The Renewal of Catholic Health Care
Formation In Christ

Monsignor Mark J. Merdian

ISBN: 978-1-711-84816-7

Printed/distributed by Amazon Kindle Direct Publishing

Cover Image: The Red Cross is the universal symbol of a hospital and it becomes the guiding image of where people go to find healing and comfort. Catholic health care in the United States is in need of renewal. Its renewal will only happen when formation in Christ becomes the guiding principle of all individuals charged with leading and those missioned in Catholic health care. The first ray coming from the cross of Christ is symbolic of the first religious whose dedication and self-sacrifice began the compassionate and healing ministry of Jesus. The second ray depicts the rapid development of Catholic health care into large health care systems sometimes without the needed formation in Christ of its leaders. The third ray illustrates that the role of leadership in Catholic health care, formerly offered by dedicated religious, must now be taken up by faith filled and well formed lay men and women in Christ who see Catholic health care as continuing the mission of Christ in our modern world. Each ray coming out of the cross of Christ touches the very heart and existence of Catholic health care, past, present and future. The rays also return to Christ who is the source of all that we do in Catholic health care. These three rays reflect the love and grace of the divine Trinity in whose image Catholic health care exists today and whose future the same Triune God must guide.

Table of Contents

Chapter 3 The New Evangelization and the Call to Mission in Catholic Health Care 51

Chapter 4 The Future of Catholic Health Care Ministry 77

Dedication

This book is dedicated to countless religious women and men who selflessly ministered to the sick, the blind, the lame in Catholic health care in the United States. Their self sacrifice and risk to bring the healing power of Christ and his love to these hurting men, women and children is a model of love for us all to imitate and carry to the next generation. It is to them and the Church's mission of Catholic Health Care that I dedicate this work.

Acknowledgments

I am grateful to many people who have made this work possible. First, I must give thanks to God for the passion he inspires within me when I talk and write about Catholic health care. Second, I want to thank Bishop Daniel Jenky, CSC for his support of and encouragement in the field of Catholic health care ministry in the Diocese of Peoria in Illinois. He has been so supportive of our care and guidance of the faith-filled and excellent hospitals already ministering within the Diocese of Peoria. I am also grateful that he allowed me the time to pursue this important topic. Next, I am grateful for my many gifted professors, especially Dr. Mark Latkovic, STD an expert in this field who encouraged, guided, and added helpful comments along the way, and to Fr. Peter Ryan, STD who offered insightful clarifications and guidance about this work. I am grateful to my many readers, proofers, and editors, namely Dr. Joseph Piccione, STD, Dr. Joseph Dockery-Jackson, PhD, Hank Wilkinson, PhD, Fr. Gerald White, and Mr. Steve Mattern. Finally, I am thankful for the support of the many mission partners whom I have collaborated with in the ministry of Catholic health care in Illinois and throughout the United States. I am also grateful for the support and encouragement I have received from individuals and parish communities I have served in while writing, especially the people of St. Pius in Rock Island, Illinois.

Foreword

"In the joy and peace of our Lord Jesus Christ I greet you and thank you for your warm welcome. This meeting gives us the opportunity to honour and give thanks to God for one of the most extensive and fundamental works of the Catholic Church in the United States, all that is embraced in the term 'Catholic health care.'" Such were the opening words of the historic 1987 meeting of Pope John Paul II and the leaders of Catholic health care in Phoenix.

A moment later the Pope added emphasis to the significance of the health care ministry. "Your health care ministry, pioneered and developed by congregations of women religious and congregations of brothers, is *one of the most vital apostolates* of the ecclesial community and *one of the most significant services* which the Catholic Church offers to society in the name of Jesus Christ."

In the nation, the surge of European immigrants in the nineteenth century brought vowed religious congregations, primarily of women, who accompanying their ethnic groups, initially founded schools, motherhouses, academies and simple hospitals. By the late nineteenth century, advances in antisepsis and anesthesia positioned these hospitals to become the natural sites of surgical advances. Through this, the vowed religious mostly sustained the workforce of the hospital.

As American healthcare became more complex through the twentieth century to an even greater level in the post-World War II era, more laypersons were hired for management roles. Those laity were "raised by the Sisters" and inculturated by the Sisters in their charism and ministry. By the dawn of the twenty-first century, Catholic healthcare was no longer the stand-alone acute care facility and becoming a continuum of care, with more persons served in the ambulatory service than acute care. And as the number of vowed religious in this work continued to decline, many religious found they were called to a "prophetic" role of formation of the next generation of leaders in an intentional manner.

It has been said that a primary responsibility of a profession, even more critical than the work before it, is to form the next generation in the profession. This is true for the healthcare professions; many Catholic hospitals are sites for medical and nursing education and residencies and they see this first hand. Formation of the next generation is obvious in the postulancy and novitiate processes of vowed religious. However, intentional formation within Catholic healthcare had something of a lag in response; operational competence expectations were always present, but perhaps there was an assumption that the inner spirit of the sponsoring congregation was always in the air and forming the culture. As the Church, we're not complete if we see ourselves solely in the good work to which we are so dedicated. St. Paul writes in 1 Cor. 13 that loves animates and is the touchstone.

Monsignor Mark Merdian's book arrives at a time of increasing intentional dedication to formation of persons, particularly leaders in American Catholic healthcare. Msgr. Merdian is not an outsider to Catholic healthcare, but a devoted liaison of the Bishop of Peoria to the ministry in the diocese, which spans central Illinois from the Iowa to the Indiana state lines. Msgr. Merdian will be heard by Catholic healthcare leaders, of course, and those dedicated to formation work, as well as by the hierarchy, to support their awareness of formation activity both underway and possible across the nation.

For many of us, the most compelling line of the *Ethical and Religious Directives for Catholic Health Care Services* is from the General Introduction, "...to see Christian love as the animating principle of health care...." Msgr. Merdian rightly draws attention to the central theological virtue of love as well as to the Holy Spirit, the gift of love, who animates all good. This study relies, in a very practical way on St. Paul's Letter to the Ephesians, 4:11, that the Spirit is in fact building up the Body of Christ with gifts to sustain the work and translate it into the future shape healthcare will take in the next decades. But do we have eyes for the work of the Spirit and availability to the Spirit so that we and our work in the Church can be actualized? A great benefit of our own time is the enhanced theological reflection on the work of the Spirit, launched in a significant way by the Second Vatican Council and *Lumen Gentium*, 12.

Msgr. Merdian layers his analysis with voices and their insights on the past and our grounding call; the challenge of the moment and practical paths to an integrated spiritual competency for this work in the future. He calls to his presentation St. Paul the Apostle on the Holy Spirit; the Second Vatican Council; Pope John Paul II; Sister Teresa Stanley; Pope Benedict; Therese Lysaught; Gerald Arbuckle; Celeste Mueller, Jack Mudd and Andre Delbecq, among others. In a truly Catholic sense, all and more, are part of our present conversation. In this book, Msgr. Merdian now joins this conversation in a robust manner, confident that we can respond to the call and sustenance of the Spirit.

Joseph J Piccione, STD, JD

Preface

Catholic health care has been a passion of mine since I began my studies for the priesthood in 1989. It became a passion because I could foresee the medical-moral field rapidly changing and I wanted to be a part of it to help guide it and influence the field. I also knew that with health care's rapid development great care and caution would have to be exercised in implementing health care decisions for persons, both Catholic and non-Catholic. Catholic health care has been instrumental in bringing about the Gospel message of Jesus. In fact, it was one of the earliest mission apostolates of the Church. Consecrated religious such as St. Angela Merici, Mother McCauley, Mother Anselma and Mother Guerin to name just a few began ministering in Catholic health care because they wanted to perpetuate Jesus' healing mission.

Although strong in its identity and legacy, Catholic health care has been adversely affected by rapid developments in the health care field. The decline in the numbers of religious leadership has affected Catholic health care and jeopardized its mission. If the Church is to sustain Catholic health care as a mission, then we must review and adapt the current structure of formation in leadership ministry.

Thus, the topic of leadership formation in Catholic health care is urgent for anyone involved in directing, overseeing, supervising or envisioning Catholic and non-Catholic health care, namely consecrated religious who are currently leading Catholic health care institutions, Sponsoring Congregations,

Catholic Health Care Boards, physicians, health care workers, bishops, and visionary lay men and women. By a Sponsoring Congregation, I am referring to the structure recognized in Church Law (Canon Law), which is a group of consecrated religious in the Church which traditionally began a Catholic hospital many years ago before it developed into the current structure it is today. Some examples of Sponsoring Congregations, especially early Congregations in the United States could include the Sisters of Mercy, the Sisters of St. Francis of the Third Order Regular or the Daughters of Charity who became then the sponsoring Congregation of the hospital or hospital system which includes other lay employees or health care institutions.

A new term from *Canon Law* or Church law, has also surfaced as a way to carry on the mission of Catholic health care without the religious sisters who once sponsored a ministry.[1] This new term, which many religious congregations have begun to apply for through Canon Law, is a *juridic person*, which can be either public or private.[2] With the decline in the number of religious, who still desire to guide their ministry of Catholic health care with the Vatican and local Bishops permission, a public juridic person can be established by the Vatican to assist in overseeing the mission of a Catholic health care institution. This canonical entity can be composed of religious sisters and lay-men and women can be the vehicle of continuing the mission originally begun by the Sisters. Although, this topic is

---

1 Sharon Holland, "Vatican Expert Unpacks Canonical JPJ Process," *Health Progress* (September-October 2011), 50-62.

2 *Code of Canon Law (Latin-English Edition), (Washington, DC: Canon Law Society of America, 1999),* Canons 113-123. See also Leonard Nelson's chapter "Catholic Hospitals and Canon Law" found in *Diagnosis Critical*, pp 90-93.

not addressed in this work, the formation of a "Juridic Person" or the group of persons entrusted with this Catholic ministry of health care is also urgent and essential as this juridic person will be charged with making important decisions for the future of this ministry of the Church.

The Lord has equipped our health care leaders with spiritual graces, charisms, and gifts to enable them to lead in the field of Catholic health care. These faith leaders are not simply running a corporation; they are fulfilling the mission of the Church by bringing the message of Jesus to those they care for in their health care settings. The spiritual works they perform affects the salvation and holiness of each person in the world redeemed by Jesus. The example of these faith-filled leaders or lack of clear religious identity and mission will either lead the health care institution forward in this mission or block the mission by focusing only on making a profit.

This book is timely and critical for understanding how to navigate the future of Catholic health care. It was originally written for an academic purpose, and has since been rewritten and revised, but I am confident it can provide the necessary guidance for those who form leaders in Catholic health care and for those who strive to lead in this complex and changing environment. The book provides practical ideas for leadership formation for those leading or those already charged with leadership in Catholic health care.

In this book, I will expound on the biblical foundations of healing and relate these foundations to the Church's development of the distinct care and respect that must be given to each human person, which incudes persons made in the image and likeness of God with a body and soul. I will describe how Saint John Paul II's theory of *Personalism* helps us to expound this rich understanding of the dignity of each human person. This Chapter will continue with a brief history of Catholic health care in the United States. What is appropriate to the topic, which I recount, is the rich history of the Sisters of the Third Order of St. Francis who came to Peoria in the late 1800's and how their mission continues the mission and ministry of Catholic health care today.

I will then describe external and internal challenges faced in Catholic health care, such as government intrusion, the issue of reproductive rights, and the challenge of financial reimbursements for Catholic health care. The internal challenges are just as serious and consist of the weakening of Catholic identity in Catholic health care, the decrease in religious leadership in our Catholic hospitals, as well as the complications which have been experienced with mergers of Catholic institutions with non-Catholic institutions.

Next, I will explore how a renewed emphasis on spiritual formation in Christ for all involved in Catholic health care can lead to a renewed evangelization in the world. This renewed and deep spiritual grounding of Catholic health care leaders and others will strengthen the mission of bringing Christ and the Faith to those in Catholic hospitals. I will discuss how the laity have been charged and equipped by God in order to fulfill this role. This equipping is not meant for personal sanctification but to support and enhance the apostolate of Catholic health care as a particular mission of the Church through the work of the laity.

Finally, lest I say all these things without entering into a plan of action to help our Catholic health care leaders and those who form them, I have written, what I consider a unique feature. I have included an introductory formation program found in Appendix A for Catholic health care leaders which shares core competencies for forming the next generation of health care leaders. This plan spans three years and offers core competencies and topics for leaders in Catholic health care. I also propose that Catholic health care institutions work with Catholic institutions of higher learning to establish educational curriculums or programs that help both institutions fulfill their mission of brining Christ to the world. I also share a template of a Retreat Module for a weekend retreat for Catholic health care leaders found in Appendix B.

The formation of Catholic health care leaders will only be fruitful when Sponsoring Congregations, executives, bishops, health care vicars, and Catholic health care leaders respond to the invitation of Jesus "come and be my disciple." By experiencing, knowing, and loving Christ at the core of one's life, then our Catholic health care leaders will be able to lead their institutions with purpose, direction, and passion.

Introduction

We value things that give meaning to our lives, whether they are gifts from our parents or an heirloom from our grandmother. We also value things from the past, not necessarily in themselves, but for what they represent. Catholic health care in the United States can be thought of in this way. For those suffering and needing healing, Catholic health care represents a gift of God's love in Jesus Christ through the Church's long-standing healing ministry to the diseased, the forgotten, the immigrant and the abandoned. Many people today still respond with nostalgia or stories of how they remembered sister so and so who cared for them in their illness at a Catholic hospital years ago.

Catholic health care is facing many external and internal challenges. As a central part of the Church's sanctifying mission, with its emphasis on the dignity of each person, who is created in the image and likeness of God, Catholic health care continues to be a light to the nations. Through a renewed emphasis on the spiritual formation of lay leaders, Jesus must be even more at the center of Catholic health care institutions and this light must be shone to all persons of the world. A Christocentric approach to the Church's two-fold mission to heal and to proclaim the kingdom of God (Mark 16:15 and Luke 24:46-48) is expressly what the Second Vatican Council, in its Dogmatic Constitution on the Church, *Lumen Gentium*, proposed:

> The term laity is here understood to mean all the faithful except those in holy orders and those in the

state of religious life specially approved by the Church. These faithful are by baptism made one body with Christ and are constituted among the People of God; they are in their own way made sharers in the priestly, prophetical, and kingly functions of Christ; and they carry out for their own part the mission of the whole Christian people in the Church and in the world.[3]

The Council Fathers recognized that the world was rapidly changing, as were Church institutions. The world of today is vastly different from the one of the mid-1960s.

Faced with a secular culture generally hostile to the Church and reflecting on the role of Catholic health care, we can ask: How will the Church continue the mission of bringing healing and holiness to Catholic health care, as the religious sisters, who so faithfully dedicated themselves to this sacred mission of the Church, continue to decline in numbers? It is a question that those in health care leadership, religious congregations and bishops, have thought and prayed about. The challenge of Catholic health care is to be a light of Christ's love in a darkened world. I would propose that Catholic health care can be transformed and sustained as a mission of the Church only if lay men and women, responding to their baptismal call from Jesus, are intentionally formed, sustained, and nourished as leaders filled with the Holy Spirit. This book will treat the above subject in four chapters, including two very important Appendixes on a module of leadership formation and a retreat for Catholic health care leaders.

Chapter 1 provides the grounding of Catholic health care ministry in the biblical references to healing from God

3 Second Vatican Council. *Lumen Gentium*, 31. Dogmatic Constitution on the Church, 1964.

as recounted in the Old Testament and those in the New Testament mentioned by Jesus. This chapter also highlights the spiritual foundation of physical and spiritual care for each human person found in Jesus' life and teaching. The caring of Jesus, the Great Physician, was shown physically and then spiritually in bringing people healing, love, care, and compassion. The incarnational presence of God's love in Jesus Christ has been carried out in the Church's ministry in the world and particularly in Catholic health care. The Catholic Church sees the inseparable unity of the whole person as foundation to theology and in particular in Catholic health care. This understanding of the unity of the body and soul in each human person means that treating individuals medically is more than just an exercise in physical healing, but a response by Jesus for the total healing of the body and soul, who is the human person with dignity and honor and meant for eternity with God.

The healing examples described in the Old Testament and the New Testament are presented and then linked to Pope St. John Paul II's personalism, which emphasizes the innate dignity of each person as a child of God. This chapter describes Catholic health care by discussing its historical development in the United States. This chapter briefly recounts the early foundations of religious orders that responded to the invitation of bishops and priests to care for the poor, the diseased, orphans, and the sick. These congregations of women religious were selfless, generous, and Spirit-led women who had consecrated themselves to the evangelical counsels of poverty, chastity, and obedience for the purpose of serving Christ in the Church. Many of them were not professionally trained in health care, but they sought to work together with lay-men and women to nurture, heal, and bring Christ's saving love to those they served. In particular, the chapter describes the missionary work that the Sisters of the Third Order of St. Francis, based in East Peoria, Illinois, undertook at the invitation of a priest who needed help caring for his people. It is a health care system that lives well the urgent call to form leaders in the true life of Jesus. Finally, this chapter reviews the mission of Catholic health care apostolate as described by the Church in documents put forth by the Holy See and the United States Bishops in the *Ethical and Religious Directives for Catholic Health Care Services* (henceforth ERD) by the United States Conference of Catholic Bishops. These directives, although containing teaching that is part of the Ordinary Magisterium or teaching office of the Church, have not been adhered to in all Catholic health care facilities.

Chapter 2 discusses the challenges to Catholic health care externally and internally. Examples are shared with the reader of external challenges facing Catholic health care, especially in the context of the culture of death. This growing culture of death has manifested itself through a rise in mercy killing laws, physician-assisted suicide, euthanasia, and unethical medical research on human embryos, to name just a few. There is also increased governmental pressure on Catholic health care to expand reproductive rights and eliminate all restrictions to those rights and to full coverage of abortion or contraceptives. This section also details some of the financial challenges being faced in Catholic health care on the federally level as well as state wide.

This chapter continues with the internal challenges many Catholic hospitals face because their longstanding Catholic culture has weakened with the steady decline of religious women and men working in Catholic health care. With the absence of women and men religious from the floors to the board rooms, Catholic health care has had to rely on the service of dedicated lay men and women who, because of their baptism in Christ, feel called to work with the religious in the Church's mission of caring for God's beloved people, especially the sick and dying. However, the formation of these lay people was accompanied by an abbreviated formation in the purpose and mission of Catholic health care. Sometimes their formation included mission and apostolate, while other times it included solely social justice concerns or how to increase the bottom line. Some religious congregations or sponsors embraced and promoted formation of their lay co-workers in the faithful discharge of their apostolate for the Church. Other health care sponsors failed to do so, did not have trained individuals, or offered misguided training which, in the end, had a negative impact on the Catholic identity of their institution. One of the last internal challenges to Catholic health care has been the impact of some early mergers where Catholic identity was not fully upheld or implemented.

Chapter 3 describes how the new evangelization, proposed by Saint John Paul II can enlighten, inspire, and inform leadership in Catholic health care in the United States. Evangelization will be discussed through the lens of St. Paul, who understood the goal of preaching the Gospel of Jesus and described that mission in the Book of *Ephesians*, especially in chapter four. This mission, begun at baptism for all the faithful, as called forth by Jesus and enumerated by St. Paul, is the foundation for all missionary activity in the Church, especially for the laity in Catholic health care. This call to health care ministry as a mission of Christ and the Church is the way in which the laity, along with all members of the Church, including the hierarchy, will serve the Lord in their brothers and sisters, especially those in need. This new understanding of leadership in Christ will allow lay health care leaders to be equipped for their future mission leadership in Catholic health care ministry with a focus on lay ministry as called forth by the Second Vatican Council.

Chapter 4 envisions the future of Catholic health care ministry and demonstrates the urgency of leadership formation. This chapter will give a list of core competencies to focus upon in ministry formation, describe the ministry leadership formation program as implemented by OSF health care in Peoria and detail how effective this type of formation program has been in forming Catholic health care leaders for the next generation of leadership in the Church's ministry. The key to renewal in Catholic health care is an enhanced, intentional, and deepened sense of belonging to Christ in the Church. A personal relation with Jesus will aid Catholic health care to flourish because lay leaders will model this experience of love in their ministry.

Lastly, this book will conclude with my hope for the future and how those various leaders formed more deeply and grounded more completely in the apostolate and ministry of Catholic health care, along with all those involved in this ministry who have been formed in Christ must play a part Catholic health care's future transformation.

Appendix A explores the future of Catholic health care as I propose new modules and the necessity of enhanced formation programs for lay men and women who are now assuming the mission and ministry of Catholic health care leadership. This chapter also reviews current programs that are being implemented to sustain and strengthen the mission of Catholic health care in the legacy of the religious sisters who began them. The leadership formation program proposes a three-year formation program with accompanying topics that will assist leaders in bringing about a deeper understanding and living of the new evangelization in the field of Catholic health care and conclude with the goal of personal faith formation of leaders, especially through a personal encounter with Jesus.

Appendix B provides a two-day ministry formation retreat for lay leaders in Catholic health care using the principles covered in this book.

When we value something, we see it as a gift and want to sustain, preserve, and protect it. Catholic health care is one of those precious gifts of the Church that needs to be strengthened. The strengthening of Catholic health care lay leaders will happen only by an increased attentiveness to well-designed, enhanced, and sustained Catholic leadership formation programs. By deepening our response to Jesus' invitation to be holy and bring that holiness to the world, Catholic health care will continue as a mission of the Church to bring God's healing to the people.

A Brief History of Catholic Health Care in the United States

The Church, after the example of Jesus, has always sought to care for the needy, especially the sick. As we have shown previously, the Church served the sick as an integral part of her mission.[4] The Church sees in the creation of the human person a being of infinite value and worth. The care of human people is closely connected to their physical and spiritual dignity. The *Ethical and Religious Directives for Catholic Health Care Sixth Edition (ERD's)*, an authoritative document approved by the United States Conference of Catholic Bishops in 2018 states: "Catholic health care has the responsibility to treat those in need in a way that respects the human dignity and eternal destiny of all."[5] The early religious recognized the dignity of each human person without regard to color, creed, or nationality. Because they viewed the person as a unity of body and soul, *both* body

---

4 John Paul II, *Motu Proprio, Dolentium Hominum* (February 11, 1985), n. 1: AAS 77 (1985), 457. In a presentation to its 27th international conference in 2013, former President of the Pontifical Council for the Pastoral Care of Health Care Workers, Cardinal Zygmunt Zimowsk, said that "The Church, adhering to the mandate of Jesus, '*Euntes docete et curate infirmos*' (Mt 10:6-8, Go, preach and heal the sick), during the course of her history, which by now has lasted two millennia, has always attended to the sick and the suffering."

5 United States Conference of Catholic Bishops, *The Ethical and Religious Directives for Catholic Health Care Service*, Fifth Edition (Washington, D.C.: 2009), 11.

1

and soul needed to be tended to in the name of Christ. Two authors succinctly comment on this dignity: "Catholic health care holds in sacred trust the healing ministry of Jesus, with its distinctive vision of the human person, the common good and the divine source and end of life."[6]

The first religious orders originated as religious associations to care for those whom the state did not attend to or provide care. The early religious found in the Corporal and the Spiritual Works of Mercy [see the Catechism of the Catholic Church paragraph 2447] the action of love, which Jesus commanded in the Gospel of Matthew (Matthew 25:35-36). The Pontifical Council for Health Care Workers also speaks clearly to the spiritual mission of the early religious:

> Faithful to the mandate received, and following the example of Christ, her Lord, who in welcoming the sick predisposed the multitudes to listening to the Word, to the conversion of lives and to believing in the Gospel, the Church over the course of the centuries "has felt strongly that service to the sick and suffering is an integral part of her mission", and not only has she encouraged among Christians the blossoming of various works of mercy, but she has also established many religious institutions within her with the specific aim of fostering, organizing, improving and increasing help to the sick.[7]

---

6 Jeanne Buckeye and Michael Naughton, "The Importance of Leadership Formation," 41.

7 The Pontifical Council for Health Care Workers, *Pastoral Care in Health and the New Evangelization for the Transmission of the Faith*, 9.

Biblical Foundations of Healing

The healing power of God is clearly evident in Sacred Scripture. The Old Testament stories of people who experienced the divine healing of God are as informative and instructive as are the stories found in the New Testament. In Exodus 23:25, we hear of God's desire to bring healing and wholeness to the nation of Israel. In 2 Kings, we read of the encounter of Naaman who is filled with leprosy and who receives healing through Elisha, the man of God (2 Kings 5:10, NAB). There is also the story of God's encounter with Tobit through the angel Raphael who is known as "one who heals" (Tobit 12:14). God's healing work of raising to life those who have died is beautifully described in 1 Kings 17:17-24, where Elijah is given power by God to bring back to life a child who is then restored to his mother.

God's healing of physical illnesses was a prefigurement of the spiritual healing that God would give through his Son, Jesus. God's power was revealed because God wanted to renew all things, the physical and the spiritual, in Christ. As Mark Latkovic writes: "These goods [of life, health, and so on] and the worthiness of the healer who ministers to them, unabashedly attested to in these passages from the Old Testament sage Sirach, are affirmed in the New Testament in the many miraculous healings performed by Jesus and His disciples."[8] God healed and brought the ultimate healing through his Son Jesus' death on the cross for our salvation.

Works of healing filled Jesus' daily life. When Jesus called his first disciples, he called them to serve as he did at the Last

---

8 Mark S. Latkovic, "The Vocation to Heal: Health Care in the Light of Catholic Faith: Scriptural, Theological, and Philosophical Reflections." *The Linacre Quarterly* 75 (1) (February 2008), 41.

Supper. "If I, therefore, the master and teacher, have washed your feet, you ought to wash one another's feet. I have given you a model to follow, so that as I have done for you, you should also do" (John 13:14-15). St. Luke continues this same understanding in Luke 22:27, "For who is greater; the one seated at table or the one who serves? Is it not the one seated at table? I am among you as the one who serves."

The Gospel of St. Luke is known as a Gospel of Healing[9], and it can be seen as such in this passage "The Spirit of the Lord is upon me, because he has anointed me to preach good news to the poor. He has sent me to proclaim liberty to the captives and recovering of sight to the blind, to set at liberty those who are oppressed..." (Luke 4:18). Jesus came to bring healing to each person he encountered, to make them whole so that the saving love of God would be experienced in each human heart. The Catechism of the Catholic Church echoes this same point, "Jesus has the power not only to heal, but also to forgive sins; he has come to heal the whole man, soul and body; he is the physician the sick have need of."[10]

Jesus' healing ministry touched the pain of each person, but it pointed to a greater reality: the healing from sin and the separation from God and others. Benedict Ashley and Kevin O'Rourke drive to the heart of the healing Jesus brought:

Jesus healed people radically by penetrating to the

---

9 St. Luke was known in the early Church as a physician who treated Christians and others out of charity and love in the name of Christ. Luke's vocation as a physician is seen in his descriptions and care of the poor, the outcast, the sick and sinners, thus it is know as the Gospel of Healing.

10 Catechism of the Catholic Church, p1503. See also the excellent theological reflection on healing and the reference to the Sacrament of Anointing of the Sick found in the Catechism, numbers 1506-1513.

spiritual core of the human personality and liberating the person from original or social sin and also from individual, personal sin, with the more superficial but real effect of healing them also psychologically and physically.[11]

Examples of that total healing can be seen, in particular, in the raising of the daughter of Jairus (Luke 8:49-56), the healing of the blind man (Mark 1:40-42), the story of the Good Samaritan (Luke 10:29-37), and the healing of the leper (Matthew 8:1-4). There are many other references to Jesus' healing and restorative grace in the New Testament. Howard Kee writes of Jesus' significant healing ministry in the Christian scriptures:

> Of the approximately 250 literary units into which the first three gospels are divided in a typical synopsis, one fifth either describe or allude to the healing and exorcistic activities of Jesus and the disciples. Of the seven "signs" reported in John to have been done by Jesus, four involved healing or restoration. Of the seventy literary units in John, twelve either describe his healing activity or refer to the signs, which he performed.[12]

Jesus didn't just bring physical healing, for Greek and Roman "healers" could do the same. No, Jesus brought much more than the healing of people's bodies; he brought forgiveness

---

11 Benedict M. Ashley and Kevin D. O'Rourke, *Healthcare Ethics: A Theological Analysis* (St. Louis, MO: The Catholic Health Association, 1989), 137.

12 Howard Kee, "Medicine, Miracle and Magic in New Testament Times," *Society for New Testament Studies*, ed. G.N. Stanton (London, UK: Cambridge University, 1986), 123.

of sin, redemption, and restoration to God the Father and to the Church as the Body of Christ.

Catholic Teaching on Care of the Person

Saint John Paul II in an address to leaders in Catholic health care wrote this about Jesus' healing: "These cures (of Jesus), however, involved more than just healing sickness. They were also prophetic signs of his own identity and of the coming of the Kingdom of God, and they very often caused a new spiritual awakening in the one who had been healed."[13] The powerful healing from sin brought with it the gifts of the Holy Spirit such as love, forgiveness, mercy, compassion, and peace. The Pontifical Council for Health Care Workers summarizes Jesus' healing ministry, which the Church continues today: "Care for the sick and activity involving healing, as is borne witness to by the Gospels, are important moments of the unique evangelization action of Jesus and a visible sign of the presence of the Kingdom of God amongst us."[14]

Treating Body and Soul

Inspired by Christ-like love and a desire to serve, women and men religious cared for the spiritual and physical needs of those no one else was willing to care for—saints and sinners alike.

---

13 John Paul II, "Address of His Holiness John Paul II to the Leaders in Catholic Health Care, Phoenix, Arizona, Monday, 14 September 1987. https://w2.vatican.va/content/john-paul-ii/en/speeches/1987/september/documents/hf_jp-ii_spe_19870914_organiz-sanitarie-cattoliche.html (accessed July 14, 2017).

14 The Pontifical Council for Health Care Workers, *Pastoral Care in Health and the New Evangelization for the Transmission of the Faith.* Editrice Velar, Gorle (BG), February: 2014, 9.

They imitated Jesus' love and compassion as commanded by him in the Gospel of Matthew: "For I was hungry and you gave me food, I was thirsty and you gave me drink… I was sick and you visited me… (Matthew 25:35-36). The early religious saw the person as an integral whole, body and soul, and both parts needed to be tended to. The ERD's clearly recognize this inseparability of the body and soul: "Modeling their efforts on the Gospel Parable of the Good Samaritan, these communities of women and men have exemplified authentic neighborliness to those in need (Lk 10:25-37)."[15] By caring for each person, regardless of his or her faith practice, the early religious gave witness to the Church's belief in the inherent dignity of the human person. This inherent dignity comes from our creation in God's image as male and female (see Genesis 1 & 2). Zeni Fox sums up this incarnational concept:

> Though in some eras religion has viewed the body with suspicion, Christian faith believes otherwise. It teaches that our human bodies are holy ground, created good by God. The Word of God dignified our bodies by becoming one of us, fully human, in our flesh. God's Spirit moves and works in the world through our bodies, which will share in Christ's glory and be raised on the last day.[16]

Of course, this innate dignity of every human person

---

15 *Ethical and Religious Directives*, General Introduction, 4.

16 Regina Bechtle, "Giving the Spirit a Home: Reflections on the Spirituality of Institutions," in *Called & Chosen: Toward a Spirituality for Lay Leaders*, ed. Zeni Fox and Regina Bechtle Lanham, MD,: Rowman & Littlefield Publishers, 2005), 102. Regina Bechtle helps one to see how the incarnation shapes all of Catholic theology as well as Catholic health care and the dignity of the human body, 99-111.

has not always been recognized or respected by cultures, governments, or those in positions of power. Throughout history, the poor, certain nationalities, particular religions, and the disenfranchised have not always received the care due them by society. Discussing this problem is beyond the scope of this work, but the Church's care for those in need follows from what was at the heart of Jesus' own healing ministry.

Today more than ever, there is a misguided effort to separate the person, understood simply as their body, from their spirit. Saint John Paul II identified the problem in his *Letter to Families* when he wrote on the topic of family life and human sexuality: "It is typical of rationalism to make a radical contrast in man between spirit and body, between body and spirit. But man is a person in the unity of his body and spirit."[17] This unnecessary separation is often experienced in the health care field where, especially at the end of life, physicians treat the dying body, but do not recognize the dignity of the soul, whose purpose is to be reunited to God. A holistic understanding of the human person must take the place of this dualistic view.

Edmund Pellegrino, the late well-known medical-moralist, states it well: "The one who is sick has a special claim on our solicitude, love and compassion, for without meeting these claims, the healer cannot truly heal."[18] As Pellegrino also

---

17 John Paul II, *Letter to Families*, February 2, 1994, no. 19. See also Michael Waldstein, *Theology of the Body* (Boston, MA: Pauline Books & Media, 2006), 43. These comments by the Pope speak to the misplaced desire of the modern culture to divide or separate the person. Acting on that desire denies the unity that we have as unique persons created by God for union with him and one another. This misguided separation is often held especially in the area of sexuality.

18 Edmund D. Pellegrino and David C. Thomasma, *The Christian Virtues in Medical Practice*, "Charity in Action: Compassion and Caring." (Washington, D.C.: Georgetown University Press, 1996), 84.

remarks, "What is at stake is the personhood of the patient."[19] A deeper understanding of the innate dignity and respect that is owed to every human person, created by God in his image, is provided in the writings and teachings of Saint John Paul II, especially in his theory of personalism.

Personalism of Saint John Paul II and its Impact on Catholic Health Care

Some would argue that personalism is not a philosophy at all[20] but rather a belief that is united by an understanding of an affirmation of the absolute value of the human person. The Stanford Encyclopedia of Philosophy defines personalism this way: "Personalism posits ultimate reality and value in personhood – human as well as (at least for most Personalists) divine. It emphasizes the significance, uniqueness, and inviolability of the person, as well as the person's essentially relational or communitarian dimension."[21]

The high dignity of human persons and their experiences, their unrepeatability, and their infinite value is what drew Saint John Paul II to personalism as a philosophy student. He saw a complementarity between the universal grounding of the philosophy of St. Thomas, which explores the essences of things in their cosmic relation with the world, and the personalistic understanding that seeks to understand the person as a unique and unrepeatable self. Personalism experienced

---

19 Pellegrino and Thomasma, *The Christian Virtues in Medical Practice*, 31.

20 Thomas D. Williams and Jan O. Bengtsson, "Personalism." *Stanford Encyclopedia of Philosophy*. https://plato.stanford.edu/entries/personalism/ (accessed November 12, 2017).

21 Ibid.

growth in France and the United States in the early part of the 20th century, but it was in Germany in the 1920s under Max Scheler, a philosopher and promoter of phenomenology, that the then Karol Wojtyla encountered and embraced it in depth. What the future Saint John Paul II found lacking in Scheler's personalism was his concept of God as the objective good, i.e., the source of truth where objective absolutes like love and goodness are realized. For Scheler, God is only an idea to be conceived of in the mind, but for Saint John Paul II, God is everything to the person and more than solely "in the mind."

Saint John Paul II's notion of personalism was influenced by his experiences under Nazism and Communist rule in Poland. During this time, the young Wojtyla was an eyewitness to the disrespect that was shown to persons as mere objects of the totalitarian state.[22] Saint John Paul II, with his deep faith in God and theological training, recognized the human person as a unique gift of God. Ronald Lawler comments: "His [Saint John Paul II's] personalism is concerned intensely with revealing the truth about persons, and the transcendent dignity of the person."[23] Saint John Paul II sets his understanding of the human person, created in God's image, within the context

---

22 Ronald D. Lawler, *The Christian Personalism of John Paul II* (Chicago, IL: Franciscan Herald Press, 1982), 6-7. This work provides a solid introduction to the early thought of John Paul II's personalism in which Fr. Lawler makes the correct statement that it is "Christian Personalism" that defines John Paul II. See also Kevin Schmiesing, "A History of Personalism," an unpublished manuscript, 21, found at http://ssrn. com/abstract=18511661. In his paper, Schmiesing presents an excellent short summary of personalism and comments on how Pope John Paul II was influenced by the world in which he lived. The Pope saw firsthand the lack of respect and the objectification that the people of his native Poland suffered under totalitarian rule.

23 Lawler, *Christian Personalism of John Paul II*, 22.

of a subject with personal experiences and freedom while also living within the plan of God as his final goal. Each human person, then, stands in relation to the gift, the other, and is called to live as a person (with body and soul) who offers his own gift of self to another in love.

As a bishop, Wojtyla had a profound impact on the Church's teaching on the dignity of the human person. His influence in the Church provided him the opportunity to assist in drafting many of the documents of the Second Vatican Council, notably the Constitution on the Church in the Modern World, *Gaudium et Spes*. This dogmatic Constitution speaks particularly of the "exalted dignity proper to the human person."[24] In *Gaudium et Spes*, John Paul II's attention to the human person in his unique and unrepeatable dignity can be clearly seen. The Constitution states, "This likeness reveals that man, who is the only creature on earth which God willed for itself, cannot fully find himself except through a sincere gift of himself."[25]

Saint John Paul II's writings also influenced the field of medical ethics as it was unfolding before him. In particular, his writings upholding the dignity of every human life and how society has an obligation to defend this life, John Paul II also referred to the various morally questionable scientific experiments in regard to blocking human life through contraception. Not only did Saint John Paul II uphold Pope Saint Paul VI's teaching in *Humanae Vitae*, but he also

---

24 *Gaudium et Spes*, 26. The Second Vatican Council saw societies' unprecedented reliance on the world, technological advancements, and secular answers as harmful, rather than relying on the truth and dignity that God had written on human hearts. The Council wanted to place the human community, created in God's image, at the core of all these human relationships.

25 *Gaudium et Spes*, 24.

continued this protection of human life through his weekly audiences and especially in his encyclical, *Veritatis Splendor,* where he writes, in affirmation of the profound unity of the human person as a body-soul composite:

> The spiritual and immortal soul is the principle of unity of the human being, whereby it exists as a whole- *'corpore et anima unus'*- as a person. These definitions not only point out that the body, which has been promised the resurrection, will also share glory. They also remind us that reason and free will are linked with all the bodily and sense faculties. The person, including the body, is completely entrusted to himself, and it is in the unity of body and soul that the person is the subject of his own moral acts.[26]

In the early 1990s, Saint John Paul II could clearly see the increasing attacks on human life. With the attacks directed at all stages of life, Saint John Paul II's theology of the body, his philosophy of personalism, and most importantly the teachings of Jesus all come to bear on the medical care of the human person. Each human person is a unique creation endowed with inviolability by God. Catholic bioethicist, Luke Gormally, comments on Saint John Paul II's teaching on human dignity and bioethics:

> The human body is integral to the human person and possesses the connatural dignity proper to persons. And respect for the dignity of the person entails respect for fundamental goods, which are integral

---

26 John Paul II, *Veritatis Splendor*, 48.

elements to the proper fulfillment of the person in his bodily reality.[27]

God uniquely creates each person with infinite value, irrespective of his or her medical condition or mental abilities. Each human life is ordered to God, the creator, in his or her body and soul. The body is not just a shell for the soul; rather it is an aspect of the person, participating in his or her dignity, and representing the person. Saint John Paul II will call the body an "icon" of the person.

Conclusion

Saint John Paul II's concept of personalism as a gift of oneself to another person, his prolific teaching on the dignity of human life, and his treatment of the human person as an integrated whole, can help us to understand the proper care of people in Catholic health care. It also reveals how the formation of lay leaders can have a profound impact on this care if they understand these concepts.

The mission of Catholic health care, as a command of Jesus through the Church, is based on the recognition of the invaluable dignity and unity of the human person in his or her body. Although Saint John Paul II articulated his anthropological truth in a remarkable way for our time, it has been true since God created people in his image. The care of the whole person, regardless of their status, became the reason why health care ministry became a mission of the Church to which we will now turn our attention.

---

27 Luke Gormally, "Pope John Paul II's Teaching on Human Dignity and Its Implications for Bioethics," *Philosophy & Medicine* 84 (2010), 12. Gormally clearly presents the dignity of the human person as described in Sacred Scripture and continued in John Paul II's theological writings.

Catholic Health Care in the United States

Jesus called many people to be his disciples and he chose specific people to follow him (Matthew 3: 12). Those who embraced the Christian Way of Jesus lived out their faith in service to others. Religious orders began by imitating Jesus and his care for others. They established communities in the Church to live out the tenets of Jesus through a life of service to others and under the authority of bishops. The Catholic Medical Association states, "In institutions of medicine that Catholics have long built and maintained – from hospitals to hospices, well-equipped offices to threadbare mission clinics – Christ as Divine Healer, Christ as the Suffering Servant has been the foundation."[28] The establishment of religious orders can be traced back to an unmet need and the Christ-like response that was called forth. In imitation of Jesus the healer, the Church in her members, especially in the lives of consecrated religious, served the sick, the suffering, plague victims, and the dying throughout her history. The early religious provided shelter for the traveler, places for the sick, and homes for orphaned children, mentally challenged adults, and the elderly. As Catholic religious orders began to expand, they became more active in health care. Leonard Nelson notes that "Catholic religious orders opened hospitals to care for the sick poor in Europe in the mid-nineteenth century, and these same

---

28 The Catholic Medical Association, "The Light Obscured: Mis-insurance and a Missing Relationship, Healthcare in America: A Catholic Proposal for Renewal," a Statement of the Catholic Medical Association, September 2004. http://www.cathmed.org/assets/files/CMA%20 Healthcare%20Task%20Force%20Statement%209.04%20Website.pdf (accessed October 16, 2017).

religious orders were invited by bishops to open hospitals in the United States."[29]

The first religious who answered the call and came to serve in the United States were the Ursuline Sisters, founded by St. Angela Merici in 1535, from Rouen, France. The Sisters, accompanied by three lay volunteers, came to work in New Orleans in 1727.[30] Sisters of Charity, also from France, became the first to staff an American hospital, the Baltimore infirmary (later to become the University of Maryland Hospital) in 1823.[31] The Sisters of Charity also served the first Catholic hospital, founded by Irish-American millionaire, John Mullanphy, in St. Louis in 1828.[32] These early religious came at the invitation of bishops, priests, and God's faithful to provide for the spiritual and physical needs of the new immigrant Church being established in the United States. Steven Rohlfs comments:

> Catholic health care in this country [the United States] can, for the most part, trace itself back to the middle and latter part of the last century. As Catholic immigrants flooded into this country by the millions, the bishops were left with the difficult responsibility of providing them with adequate pastoral care.[33]

Faithful religious dedicated their entire lives—, through the Evangelical Counsels of poverty, chastity, and obedience

---

29 Nelson, *Diagnosis Critical*, 84.

30 Margaret M. McGuinness, *Called to Serve: A History of Nuns in America* (New York, NY: New York University Press, 2013), 7.

31 Kauffman, *Ministry & Meaning*, 33-34.

32 Ibid., 51-52.

33 Rohlfs, *The Experience of Catholic Health Care*, 3.

(and some Orders with more specific charisms)—to care for the poor, the indigent, orphans, and the infirm. One thinks today of the Missionaries of Charity, founded by Saint Teresa of Calcutta, whose charism calls them to care for the poorest of the poor and for those who are dying. Another is the Hawthorne Dominicans, whose ministry is to those dying of cancer. These religious orders filled an urgent need and responded to Jesus' call to love one's neighbor. In doing so, they fulfilled the mission of the Church to bring health care to those in need.

Christopher Kauffman, a noted historian of Catholic health care in the United States, comments:

> Though there were priests, sisters, brothers and lay people ministering to the sick in their private homes throughout the nineteenth and into the twentieth century, this study focuses primarily on the public places where Religious Communities responded to the physically and mentally ill, in peace and in war, in times of pestilence and economic crisis, in urban centers, rural towns, and on the expanding frontiers. They nursed in ethnic Catholic enclaves and in Protestant areas of the South and West, and in hospitals maintained by physicians, cities, counties, states, mining companies, railroads, and by their own orders. While the parish, school and diocese have a public presence only the hospital is inherently a public place; here Catholics ministered to the physical, mental, emotional, and spiritual needs of people representing the entire spectrum of religious and secular traditions. Because the nurses in these public places were committed to the vowed life as sisters,

their prayer life and nursing ministry developed in an atmosphere of interdependence.[34]

Kauffman continues:

> Their rule of life may have separated private and public roles, but in fact they brought their ministry to prayer in chapel and their private life was frequently embodied in ministry. Theirs was an activist missionary spirituality that tended to be based on a positive appreciation of human experience rather than on its denial.[35]

The growth of Catholic health care, and its service at the invitation of bishops and pastors in the early pioneer days of the United States, mirrored the expansion experienced throughout the United States. In 1872, there were about 75 Catholic hospitals; by 1910, there were 400.[36] This increase was also reflected in the first Catholic nursing college in 1886 in Springfield, Illinois, which provided professional training not only for religious, but also for the laity who were being associated with the sisters in caring for the sick, the diseased, and the dying. The sisters and those they sought to associate with them, especially lay-women and men, centered their ministry on bringing their patients closer to Jesus. Giving

---

34 Kauffman, *Ministry & Meaning*, 1.

35 Ibid.

36 Gottemoeller, Doris, "Catholic Institutional Ministries: Their History and Legacy," in *Called & Chosen: Toward a Spirituality for Lay Leaders*, ed. Zeni Fox and Regina Bechtle Lanham, MD,: Rowman & Littlefield Publishers, 2005), 60. See also Wikipedia, "Catholic sisters and nuns in the United States." https://en.wikipedia.org/wiki/Catholic_sisters_and_nuns_in_the_United_States (accessed November 20, 2017).

them hope and encouragement in their time of need allowed the sisters to eventually prepare them for death and resurrected life in Christ. That mission continues today.

The Sisters of the Third Order of St. Francis of Peoria, Illinois

The Sisters of St. Francis of the Third Order Regular began their ministry as a religious congregation founded in Germany. Their charism included care of the sick, especially children who were abandoned or surrounded by extreme poverty. The Sisters, as well as the Church in Germany, began to suffer religious persecutions in the middle of the 1800s. At the invitation of a priest in Iowa, 12 Sisters arrived in Iowa City, Iowa, in 1875. Sister Alice O'Rourke, a historian of the Diocese of Peoria in Illinois wrote: "Father Bernard Baak of St. Joseph Parish, Peoria, heard of a group of Franciscan Sisters who had taken refuge in America to escape the 'May Laws' of Bismarckian Germany and had settled in Iowa."[37] The Sisters traveled to cities in the area begging for money for the children in the orphanage that they had started and encountered Father Bernard Baak who spoke to them of the need of the German Catholic community in Peoria. They were granted permission to leave Iowa and began their new mission in Peoria.

In 1876, the Sisters began their ministry of Catholic health care in Peoria. The Sisters cared for the sick and those living in poverty according to the ideal of St. Francis and all Franciscans. In 1877, the new Bishop of the Diocese of Peoria, John Lancaster Spalding, recommended that the Sisters form a new Order and establish it as a Diocesan Order. On July

---

37 Alice O'Rourke, *The Good Work Begun: Centennial History of Peoria Diocese* (Peoria, IL: R.R. Donnelley & Sons Company, 1970), 31.

16, the ten Sisters took the name of The Sisters of the Third Order of St. Francis. The Sisters bought property on a bluff of the city. 1878 saw extensive renovations to the home where they first started proving health care, and St. Francis Hospital opened with 35 patient beds. As their ministry expanded in the area, a north wing was added, almost doubling the number of beds. Along with this second expansion came the extension of their apostolate to the surrounding communities that were burgeoning because of river traffic and industrial growth. The hospital continued to experience growth through the generosity of donors and another wing was added in 1890. The main portion of the hospital was built in 1901 and then another in 1942. St. Francis Hospital pioneered Catholic health care in the tri-county area and remains a faith-centered and mission-driven apostolate of the Church.

The Sisters, realizing that inviting lay men and women in their work would allow them to continue the apostolate of Catholic health care when the number of Sisters declined in the future, wisely began a ministry leadership formation program (MLFP) in the early 1980s. Since its inception, inspired by the vision and example of Jesus, St. Francis Medical Center in Peoria has continued the Church's ministry of Catholic health care. The Sisters also recognized the need to form lay-men and women in a truly Catholic ethos so that the hospital would continue as a ministry of the Church.

The Mission and Ministry of the Catholic Health Care Apostolate

The mission of Catholic health care continued to expand and its mission field grew. John Gallagher quotes Daniel Sulmasy regarding Catholic health care's spiritual mission:

In caring for the sick, in caring acts of love toward one's neighbor, one also loves Jesus. The message of the beatitudes is the message of the Good Samaritan. There is an inherent link between love of neighbor and love of God. This is the unifying religious or theological element. The primary rationale for the American Catholic health care ministry is the religious conviction that loving and serving the sick is an embodiment of what it means to love God.[38]

These early religious who came to the United States understood the invitation to serve the poor, outcast, and diseased so that the love of God, which they experienced, could be shared with those in need. As Rohlfs states regarding the importance of religious identity:

It was precisely these supernatural qualities that distinguished Catholic health care from other types of medical care. But the "specific difference" in Catholic health care lay with the sisters, or more precisely with the faith and spirituality they exuded.[39]

The Church developed from a ministry to immigrants to a recognized and robust ministry of service that expanded to

---

38 John A. Gallagher, "Discerning the Future of the American Catholic Health Care Ministry," *The National Catholic Bioethics Quarterly* Vol. 13, Issue 2, (Summer 2013), 267. Gallagher references the theme of Christ-like love that is central to Catholic health care because Jesus came to restore us to the love of the Father and Spirit through his saving death. See also Daniel P. Sulmasy's article, "Without Love, We Perish," *Health Progress* 90 (4) (July-August 2009): 30-36,

39 Rohlfs, *The Experience of Catholic Health Care*, 3.

reach all parts of the United States. The Dominican Benedict Ashley comments on this expansion in health care:

> Catholic hospitals and long term care facilities were founded principally by religious orders of sisters and brothers to give healthcare to the neglected and, especially in areas where Catholicism was not the chief religion, as a means to witness to the ethical and spiritual aspects of healthcare in accordance with Catholic values. Healthcare has always been considered an apostolate of the Church, whether offered in the home or in a more formal institution.[40]

John Gallagher also speaks to this advancement of the mission:

> It is part of the essence of Catholicism to organize itself as a Church into an institutional structure, both the hierarchical Church as well as its core ministries of health, education and charity. The mission and ministries of the Church have historically and contemporaneously been organized into institutional settings rather than through the efforts of individuals.[41]

The Church continued to advance the mission of Jesus, realizing that through the care of persons, her mission of bringing the love of Christ to all could be accomplished. As Rohlfs again comments, "For an apostolate to be truly effective, those ministered to must sense the presence of God in those

---

40 Ashley and O'Rourke, *Healthcare Ethics*, 136.

41 Gallagher, "Discerning the Future of the American Catholic Health Care Ministry," 268.

carrying out the apostolate."[42] The Church saw in this mission a way to help those in need to see Jesus as the ultimate source of healing.

According to statistics compiled by the Catholic Health Association in January of 2017, there are 649 Catholic hospitals in the United States that admitted nearly 5 million people, with 105 million outpatient visits, 20 million emergency room visits, and 527,000 deliveries of babies. One in six patients in the United States is cared for in a Catholic hospital. Catholic health care systems and facilities are present in all 50 states providing acute care, skilled-care nursing, and other services, including hospice, home health, assisted living, and senior housing.[43] The impact of Catholic health care is vast and far-reaching and has a marked influence in the spiritual and medical care of people.

Conclusion

The Church desires to include all people in the healing mission of Catholic health care. This mission, once entrusted to consecrated religious, will continue only with the involvement of lay men and women who understand Jesus' call to be his disciple, from the Sisters of St. Francis in Peoria to countless other Orders who gave so generously in Christ to make the visible love of God known in the sick and suffering. As the mission of Catholic health care continued to expand in the modern world, the leaders in Catholic health care realized the call to share that invitation with others, especially in the ministry of Catholic health care.

42 Rohlfs, *The Experience of Catholic Health Care*, 4.

43 Catholic Health Association, *Facts-Statistics: Catholic Health Care in the United States* (Updated January 2017). https://www.chausa.org/about/about/facts-statistics (accessed November 26, 2017).

CHAPTER 2

Challenges to Catholic Health Care

External Challenges to Catholic Health Care

One has only to read news articles or listen to reports about Catholic health care to grasp the external threats facing it. There have been blatant attacks by individuals, private organizations, and government regulations. These attacks seem to be aimed at destroying or severely reducing the influence of Catholic hospitals. Benedict Ashley O.P. and Kevin O'Rourke O.P. reflect on these external dangers to the Church's mission:

> Today in the United States, the dominance of secular humanism as a philosophy of life has so influenced and pressured the operation of such Catholic institutions that many wonder whether these institutions are any longer Catholic and are able to be conducted as an apostolic endeavor. [44]

The Catholic Church is called to sanctify the world around her, and she does this especially by assisting people in their most serious moments of need. Pope Pius XII also recognized this necessity. He boldly wrote and spoke on the topic of the medical–moral issues facing the Church and world in the mid-20th century. He addressed the topic in his famous address to

---

44 Ashley and O'Rourke, *Healthcare Ethics*, 136.

anesthesiologists in 1957.[45] Pius XII spoke of the importance of preserving life and yet acknowledged that life is a gift from God and is meant to return to him. The basic moral principles that have guided all Catholics in living a moral life began to be defined more precisely in the context of medical ethics, as medical science became more exact as medicine and its treatments rapidly advanced. As the ERD states:

> Throughout the centuries, with the aid of other sciences, a body of moral principles has emerged that expresses the Church's teaching on medical and moral matters and has proven to be pertinent and applicable to the ever-changing circumstances of health care and its delivery.[46]

Cognizant of the changing face of Catholic health care in the United States, with its many challenges, the Church continues its commitment to both the physical and spiritual healing of all who come to her.

Merger Watch, an initiative of the American Civil Liberties Union (ACLU), has been vehemently opposed to the moral stance of the Catholic Church in Catholic health care and Catholic social services. It published a report calling for the removal of all federal support from Catholic health care facilities. "Miscarriage of Medicine," released in December 2013, states in the introduction:

> In short, this report reveals how Catholic hospitals have left far behind their humble beginnings as facilities

---

45 Pope Pius XII, "Address to an International Congress of Anesthesiologists," http://www.lifeissues.net/writers/doc/doc_31resuscitation.html (accessed on November 26, 2017).

46 *Ethical and Religious Directives*, Preamble, 1.

established by orders of nuns and brothers to serve the faithful and the poor. They have organized into large systems that behave like businesses — aggressively expanding to capture greater market share — but rely on public funding and use religious doctrine to compromise women's health care. We make recommendations about how to ensure Catholic restrictions do not interfere with patients' rights and protect access to comprehensive reproductive health care.[47]

The report goes on to state that because Catholic health care receives federal funding, Catholic health care should be required to provide a full range of reproductive and other medical services, even those that the Catholic Church deems immoral. What this report insinuates is that Catholic health care is operating as a business more than charity care as it first began. With the current culture of payer mix and the cost of medical technology along with insurance requirements and government regulations, Catholic hospitals have been forced to compete in this competitive market while being faithful to and carrying on its religious mission. In the 1980's there was pressure from the government and insurance providers to hold down costs based on payer mix. As Leonard Nelson remarks in his book *Diagnosis Critical*, "And, in the private sector, Catholic hospitals must compete in order to remain competitive in their

---

47 Lois Uttley and Sheila Reynertson of the Merger Watch Project, and Lorraine Kenny and Louise Melling of the American Civil Liberties Union. Merger Watch: "The Growth of Catholic Hospitals and the Threat to Reproductive Healthcare," (New York: Merger Watch, 2013). See the number of reports that they have written against Catholic health care at http://www.mergerwatch.org/mergerwatch-publications/. Also see "Why is the A.C.L.U. targeting Catholic Hospitals?" in *America*, May 31, 2017 by Stephanie Slade.

pricing structures when negotiating health plans."[48] The truth must be made know that any Federal funding which Catholic health care receives assists in its mission of providing charity care and care in general to ill populations of people, whether in inner city neighborhoods or rural settings. A Catholic hospital must operate with revenue so that it can provide services to the poor and needy. Or as one religious sister used to remark, "No margin no mission."

The purpose of this report, and many others like it, is to discredit Catholic health care by appealing to the emotions of the American public. In this way, the ACLU hopes to continue to turn the culture against Catholic health care ministry by claiming it limits the rights of women and men.

Catholic health care can point to its 2000-year-old legacy of care for all patients, especially women, as the reason for its continued support. Leonard Nelson describes the struggle between the culture of life and the culture of death, an obvious reference to Saint John Paul II's Encyclical, *Evangelium Vitae*.[49] Nelson states that the Catholic mission of health care is in grave danger due to "a confluence of powerful environmental forces."[50] These powerful forces are as cultural, religious, economic, and political, and they are converging in such a way

---

48 Leonard J. Nelson, *Diagnosis Critical: The Urgent Threats Confronting Catholic Health Care*. (Huntington, Indiana: Our Sunday Visitor, 2009), 87.

49 See in particular numbers 12, 19, and 28, which describe the two opposing cultural trends. Pope John Paul II describes the culture of death, which rejects many life principles and encourages a focus on self-preservation regardless of others in need in *Evangelium Vitae*, 29.

50 Nelson, *Diagnosis Critical*, 9.

that they are affecting the very life and goodness of Catholic health care.[51]

There are numerous external challenges facing the delivery of Catholic health care some of which are too expansive for this work. I will describe a few external challenges that do impact the moral mission of Catholic health care and its inability or hampering of its Catholic mission.

Governmental Challenges

In the early 1970's there were many changes to how the federal government should treat Catholic hospitals that had for years prior operated according to Catholic moral teaching without question. A new wave of legislation wanting to respect the plurality of belief along with new laws regarding abortion and reproductive rights began to emerge. Many conscience protection laws were introduced and approved as a way of recognizing the law of abortion and the long-term respect and rights that were afforded to Catholic health care institutions who had been operating and caring for the poor and needy of this country without charge to the government since their inception in the United States.

In March 2010, President Barak Obama signed into law the Affordable Care Act. Although the Catholic Church

---

51 Nelson, *Diagnosis Critical*, 9. He starkly describes the reality of what is being faced in our culture and states that the crux of the issue is contraception and abortion on demand. Chapters 11 and 12 (pp. 151-174) cover these topics in detail. Catholic health care, as well as statements by the Catholic Church, has always held these life issues to be among the "non-negotiables." See Pope John Paul II, *Evangelium Vitae*, March 25, 1995, especially no. 62 and 13-16, as well as the *Ethical and Religious Directives for Catholic Health Care Services,* (see chapter 4 on Beginning of Life issues).

believes people have a right to basic health care[52] and strongly advocated for this in the federal health care bill, the Church could not support certain immoral practices required within the regulations. Under the ACE, all health care facilities, including Catholic ones, are required to provide contraceptives to any patients regardless of faith practice. Certain narrow exemptions are provided, e.g., for houses of worship, but not for religiously affiliated institutions such as Catholic hospitals or soup kitchens. The ACA does not grant conscience protections. After hundreds of years of civil protection in the United States, that protection was removed. The U.S. Bishops, Little Sisters of the Poor, and many Catholic hospitals and other institutions of the Church battled this law. The lawsuit filed by the Little Sisters of the Poor fought this injustice on the grounds that providing funding for contraceptive services in their insurance policy or simply signing off on it would make them morally complicit. They won an injunction against the federal government in not having to provide or even participate in this immoral action. More lawsuits would follow, repeating the same objection on moral grounds by Catholic and non-Catholic entities.[53] With

---

52 See *Pacem in Terris* (June 3, 1963), where Pope John XXIII states in no. 11 that all people created in God's image with inalienable dignity have the "right to food, clothing, shelter, medical care…". Pope Francis, in an address to the Doctors of Africa (May 10, 2016), wrote that "Health is not a consumer good but a universal right, so access to health services cannot be a privilege." See also the *Catechism of the Catholic Church*, no. 2288, as well as *The Ethical and Religious Directives for Catholic Health Care Services*, Part One.

53 The Hobby Lobby case of a Christian ("closely held") employer who refused to provide contraceptive services is most notable and helped to change the tide. See *Burwell v. Hobby Lobby Stores*, ruling on June 30, 2014. https://www.oyez.org/cases/2013/13-354 (accessed October 2, 2017).

the election of a new president in 2016, the federal mandate was rescinded by an Executive Order. Most likely, this threat will become a reality in the next election cycle. The battles against the secular culture are still being waged, especially in states requiring Catholic hospitals to provide contraceptives, sterilizations, and referrals for abortion.

Actions by the government at the state level also pose challenges to Catholic health care. For example, in January 2017, the Right of Health Care Conscience Act was passed by the Illinois legislature, requiring all health care facilities and those facilities that support pregnancy to provide in writing information regarding where to reasonably obtain abortion and contraceptive services. Through the Illinois Catholic Conference, a lobbying arm of the Illinois Bishops, the law was vehemently opposed. Despite this opposition, the law was passed. In July 2017, an Illinois federal judge granted a preliminary injunction prohibiting the state from enforcing the law while it is being argued in the courts.

Most recently, a bill was introduced by Representative Kelly Cassidy, a long-term proponent of abortion rights from Chicago, to remove and repeal all restrictions to abortion and abortion services in Illinois in House Bill 2465 in February of 2019. This proposed bill has many co-sponsors and is seemingly part of a concerted plan by organizations throughout the United States to enshrine into State Law abortion on demand. One only has to look at the rapid passage of these laws in others states in the fall of 2018 and 2019 to see the goal of particular individuals that abortion laws, irrespective of conscience rights be demolished and put asunder.

Reproductive Rights Challenges

As has been mentioned, reproductive rights for women, has been a hotly contested issue since the Roe v Wade Supreme Court decision in 1973. According to a website dedicated to the topic of law and reproductive rights, the article states:

> Historically, reproductive rights in the U.S. has seen many controversies due to the moral, ethical, and religious undertones of birth control, abortion, and family planning. Today, the subject of reproductive rights continues to be an emotionally and politically charged issue, especially in light of new technologies and recent laws. [54]

Reproductive rights covers a whole range of issues, too many to be properly covered in this book. Reproductive rights normally refers to what particular groups consider the right to kill an unborn child in the womb, a right to chemically kill a child in the womb through various types of contraceptives, the right to mutilate one's otherwise healthy reproductive organs by a tubal ligation or vasectomy for men. It also includes the whole range of topics including when does life begin, having an abortion right up to the moment of birth, or even some proponents in politics and education whether a child who is born can be killed up to two months after birth?

Although women are naturally able to bear children the question of men's rights in reproduction also enters in. Although men's reproductive rights are not often discussed and were glossed over by Court arguments, especially in Roe v Wade

---

54 Family Law. https://family.findlaw.com/reproductive-rights/what-are-reproductive-rights-.html. Accessed on March 18, 2019.

of 1973, it is nonetheless an important matter to be addressed. Another moral consideration of external challenges to Catholic health care is the topic of sex reassignment surgeries. Although it often is something surgically done in the later years of one's life, what is to prevent parents requesting that the biological sex of the child be altered before or after birth.

The issue of reproductive rights will continue to be a rallying cry for those who claim that Catholic hospitals, because they receive federal funds, should be required to provide what is legally permissible, especially in the area of contraceptive and abortive services. What Catholic health care would hold, is that within its walls, because of religious protection it can refuse these types of treatments and transfer the patient to another facility who will perform these procedures.

Financial Challenges

Another sobering external challenge for Catholic health care comes from the lack of financial reimbursements to Catholic facilities. All hospitals receive funding from third party participants for Medicare and Medicaid programs. Hospitals also receive payments from insurance companies who insure patients. For patients that do not have health insurance, Medicare and Medicaid helps to bridge that financial gap for health care facilities. Many Catholic hospitals depend upon a portion of government funding in order to operate. David Archer surmised that without government-funded programs, Catholic health care facilities would be greatly burdened. He writes, "The complexities and interrelationships of strategic, financial, and operational facets of hospitals make it very difficult if not impossible to operate without government reimbursement and Medicare certification."[55] Nelson states it bluntly, "Catholic health care leaders acknowledge that the passage of legislation linking the receipt of federal funds to the provision of reproductive services prohibited by the ERD's will effectively destroy Catholic health care."[56] The lack of sustainable reimbursements in Catholic health care affects not just Catholic hospital, but public hospitals as well.

Many Catholic hospitals, and other small public hospitals, are not flush with extra capital and often find it financially challenging to operate on such slim margins. With its continued service to the poor, the underinsured, the uninsured—and Pope Francis has often commented about this great responsibility of the Church to care for such individuals in our Catholic institutions—Catholic health care is very much dependent on reimbursement dollars.[57] The financial complications have resulted from big insurance entering the picture. The majority of health care was provided by the early religious either free of charge or with minimal payment by those receiving treatment. As health care continued to expand in this country insurance claims required by our government were paid for medical

---

55 David L. Archer, "Will Catholic hospitals survive without government reimbursements?" *The Linacre Quarterly* 84 (1) (2017), 24. See his article regarding federal and state funding. Although his article references the State of Tennessee, his points about the lack of federal funding and Medicare certification for Catholic hospitals is very clear.

56 Nelson, *Diagnosis Critical*, 12.

57 See Ron Hamel's article, "A 'Disruptor' for Catholic Health Care and Ethics?" in *Health Progress* (September-October 2014) on how Catholic health care can include justice for the poor more readily in their outlook, care, and service. Hamel asks the question, are we doing enough to care for the poor in Catholic health care?

services, thus the financial conundrum of dependency ourselves in today in the area of Catholic health care.

Medicaid reimbursement funding remains a major issue of contention today in many hospital boardrooms. According to US News, Illinois is one of the top ten states in Medicaid spending as a state, along with New Jersey, New York, Michigan and a host of other states. In other words, the amount the State of Illinois spends to assist the poor and handicap is in the top ten of US Cities. Although Illinois spending is in the top ten, Illinois also has one of the largest totals of individuals enrolled in Medicaid, totaling over 3 Million. In numbers that means that 1 out of every 4 persons is on Medicaid in Illinois. With the large number of individuals receiving funded medical care, this leaves very little for reimbursements to hospitals.[58]

The crux of the issue is the lack of reimbursements paid back to the hospitals or medical centers that are caring for all these patients. Although the State may spend a large portion of their budget $19.3, according to the article, the State of Illinois is only being reimbursed $3252.00 per beneficiary, the lowest in the nation. Surrounding states around Illinois, namely Iowa, Wisconsin, Missouri, Michigan and Indiana are spending over double what Illinois spends per beneficiary.[59] Of the five states bordering Illinois, Missouri spends the highest

58 Danny Chun, Illinois Hospital Association, "Illinois is Getting Shortchanged: Federal Contribution Per Medicaid Beneficiary 2015." Found at https://www.team-iha.org/advocacy-policy/state-issues/advocacy-tab-(1)/illinois-is-getting-shortchanged (accessed on May 2, 2019).

59 Illinois Hospital Association. "Illinois is Getting Short-changed." Federal Contribution Per Medicaid Beneficiary 2015 found at https://www.team-iha.org/advocacy-policy/medicaid (accessed on April 28, 2019).

amount of dollars per beneficiary at $6447.81 compared to Illinois' $3252.00. That is over double the amount. This money that is spent per beneficiary is not being reimbursed either fully and even the timing of reimbursement can be anywhere from 6 months to over a year. Hospitals, both Catholic and non-Catholic are finding this a serious financial strain.

A case in point is how the State of Illinois spends on average less than seventy cents per one dollar in reimbursement, while other states, such as Iowa, Indiana, and Wisconsin provide double that amount.[60] Many Illinois hospitals, both Catholic and non-Catholic are not receiving fair payment from the state of Illinois for reimbursements of Medicaid patients who are on government subsidies, thus another financial challenge. In fact, Illinois is now ranked as the lowest in Medicaid matching rates in the country according to the Illinois Hospital Association.[61] In Illinois, Catholic health care has been hit particularly hard because the State of Illinois was without a budget for two years, FY 2015-2017, and reimbursements were delayed during this period and sometimes non-existent.

Another financial challenge is Catholic hospital-funded pension plans. Some employees, encouraged by big unions or organizations trying to limit the moral impact of Catholic health care in particular states, have challenged Catholic health care's employee pension plans because they currently are exempt under ERISA (Employee Retirement Income Security Act of 1974), which permits Catholic health care institutions to manage their own retirement programs without including

---

60 Illinois Hospital Association, 2017. *What's at Stake?* Found at https://www.ihatoday.org/uploadDocs/1/2017federaladvocacyagenda.pdf

61 Ibid.

payment for any immoral services provided within the program and without government intrusion. These lawsuits contend that Catholic hospitals are not churches and are therefore not entitled to exemptions, as are Catholic parishes. However, Catholic health care is a *mission* of the Church and is not limited by buildings with steeples or bells. Mark Chopko, a long-time attorney who represents the Catholic Health Association, asked the question in regard to this issue, "What is the Church?" He stated, "In the Catholic understanding of the term, church is more than a steepled building and always was. Health care is essential and integral to the church's self-understanding of how to minister to a hurting world."[62] The question of what constitutes an apostolate or ministry of the Church is really at the core of this lawsuit. Chopko goes on to deftly argue:

> Religious orders established their ministries as expressions of the church's work; and having received permission of church authorities, healthcare sponsors are assured that their work is authentically Catholic and will remain so until the church decides otherwise, a point beyond the ability of any secular court to adjudicate. To hold otherwise would both impermissibly invade religious autonomy and jeopardize the Catholic ministries that operate beyond the walls of steepled buildings.[63]

---

62 Julie Minda, "Dozens of faith-based providers targeted in pension lawsuits." *Catholic Health World*, October 1, 2016. https://www.chausa.org/publications/catholic-health-world/article/october-1-2016/dozens-of-faith-based-providers-targeted-in-pension-lawsuits (accessed on October 2, 2017).

63 Ibid.

When the Church was engaged in Catholic health care, she served her poor and needy without government reimbursement for hundreds of years. It wasn't until insurance companies and forced government insurance programs that Catholic health care began to receive governmental funding on a state and federal level. It was a matter of justice that the very patients needing care were also people of the United States whom the government also had an obligation to care for. As funding models continued to develop, Catholic health care continued to receive payment for patients through insurance rather than federal funding, except for those who could not pay. Medicaid and Medicare then became the dominant program of reimbursement for many poor persons who did not have insurance or who were unable to afford it, but yet who needed to be cared for and treated. So this issue of federal funding could also be considered a matter of justice, which federal and state governments must provide funding for those in need that are served in Catholic health care.

Conclusion

While I could continue to cite fact after fact of the serious financial crisis facing health care institutions, in particular Catholic health care, suffice it to say, the current references allow us to see that these external challenges may become too burdensome to continue Catholic health care in the future. However, perhaps even more alarming are the challenges that Catholic health care is facing in its future leaders and in faithfulness to its Catholic identity. These issues are addressed in the next chapter.

Internal Challenges to Catholic Health Care

Quality leadership is a key to the success of any organization, and that is true for Catholic health care, too. Strong and visionary leadership helps a hospital, parish, school or business organization thrive. The internal challenge for Catholic health care today must begin with the question, "Will there be deeply committed followers of Jesus and visionary leaders to navigate the future and provide leadership of Catholic health care ministry as a mission of the Church?" The Catholic Health Association (CHA), based in St. Louis, Missouri has completed extensive studies about health care leadership. In a poignant article on the challenges facing Catholic health care leaders, Sr. Teresa Stanley writes,

> The formation of sponsors — both religious and lay — is an important issue in the continuation of sponsored ministry of Catholic institutions. As this ministry continues to evolve, and as sponsoring groups determine how best to prepare new sponsors to undertake the roles and responsibilities involved, might this not be a good time to think about ways to pool the ministry's collective wisdom on formation?[64]

Some, including Sr. Teresa, say that the formation of leaders in Catholic health care is the single most important issue facing Catholic health care today. She goes on to state, "The formation and education of lay leaders (and also of new congregational leaders who assume the sponsor role) is a

---

64 Teresa Stanley, "Can the Ministry Collaborate to Form the 'Next Generation' of Sponsors?" *Health Progress* (January-February 2007), 12.

concern many place at the forefront of these challenges."[65] To understand more clearly the reasons for these challenges to leadership in Catholic health care, let's look at how we arrived at this juncture.

The Decrease of Religious Sisters in Catholic Health Care

Catholic hospitals continued to expand and grew at a rapid pace and so did religious orders. In 1840 in the United States, there were 900 Sisters from 15 Communities; in 1900, there were 50,000 Sisters from 170 Communities and in 1930 there were 135,000 Sisters from 300 different Orders.[66] The number of religious in the United States peaked in 1965 when there were 180,000 religious.[67]

---

65 Ibid., 12. Teresa Stanley identifies the pressing need for ongoing formation in mission development for lay leaders in Catholic health care. She also sees the need for sponsors, i.e., religious sisters and board members, to have formation in the complicated moral complexities of care they will be asked to fulfill in the future. The Congregation for the Doctrine of the Faith recognizes the sacred role of boards and the moral responsibility they play in seeing that Catholic health care remains faithful to its mission from Jesus. See the CDF's document, *Some Principles for Collaboration with non-Catholic Entities in the Provision of Healthcare Services* (February 17, 2014). See also comments by Germain Grisez in *The Way of the Lord Jesus: Difficult Moral Questions,* Volume 3 (Quincy, IL): Franciscan Press, 1997), 391-402. Question 87: "How far may Catholic hospitals cooperate with providers of immoral services?"

66 James M. O'Toole. *The Faithful: A History of Catholics in America* (Cambridge, MA: Harvard University Press, 2008),104. See also "Catholic sisters and nuns in the United States," Wikipedia, https://en.wikipedia.org/wiki/Catholic_sisters_and_nuns_in_the_United_States (accessed October 16, 2017).

67 J.J. Zeigler, "Nuns Worldwide." Catholic World Report (May 12, 2011),

With the decrease of consecrated religious Sisters in Catholic health care to about 56,000 in 2010, many religious who formerly ran multi-million dollar hospitals were functioning only on a board level or serving in pastoral care in the hospitals they once led.[68] Most lay administrators had worked with these religious sisters who were visionary, committed to the people they were called to serve and were well versed in understanding the spiritual healing of Christ as central to the mission of the hospital. The focus on the spiritual care and sacramental presence remained strong for a number of years even with the continued presence of the religious in administrative roles, but the landscape in Catholic health care was beginning to change. The once palpable feeling of knowing one was in a Catholic institution could no longer be clearly perceived.

The Lack of Leadership Formation in Catholic Health Care Ministry

The first lay hospital presidents were closely supported and guided by the religious. The continued influence of the sisters' original charism, which they brought to bear on their ministry from the life of the Church, kept the Catholic identity and mission strong. However, as the number of consecrated religious declined, their influence was diminished. What most religious founders and sponsors failed to perceive was how their lack of formation of incoming lay leaders would impact the future identity of Catholic health care. An article on the handing on of this identity through formation sums it up well, "What they (the founders or sponsors) overestimated

---

68 McGuinness, Called to Serve, 179.

was the capacity for successive generations of leaders to 'catch' the mission simply by association."[69] Formation is not always caught by succeeding generations, it also must be taught. Thus the weakening of the Catholic identity and mission of Catholic health care was experienced with the departure of the religious sisters, the lack of formation programs for incoming leaders to inculcate the mission, the rapidly changing landscape of Catholic health care, and the financial stresses of the market. Steven Rohlfs sums it up well:

> Today, lay employees in Catholic hospitals still look upon the sisters as the guardians of a great legacy. Reflecting on the parameters of this legacy will show us not only the limits of our efforts, but may well challenge us to go far beyond what we are doing at present to pass on the vision and values of our sister sponsors.[70]

Leadership in Catholic health care has changed dramatically in less than a generation, and this can especially be seen in leadership positions. John O. Mudd, a senior leader in Catholic health care, writes: "Forty years ago most of the presidents of Catholic hospitals in the United States were Catholic women religious. Today, those hospitals are nearly all led by lay people, mostly men, a large number of whom are not Catholic."[71] While the experience of working alongside the religious had been instructional in strengthening the mission of

---

69 Jeanne Buckeye and Michael Naugton, "The Importance of Leadership Formation," *Health Progress* (March-April 2008), 39.

70 Steven P. Rohlfs, "Dye, Not Paint: Issues in Catholic Identity," *Ethics & Medics* (March 1997), Volume 22, Number 3, 1.

71 John O. Mudd, "From CEO to Mission Leader," *Health Progress* (September-October 2005), 25.

Catholic health care, intentional leadership and personal faith formation of the lay faithful is a key to its future. On this point, Peter J. Giammalvo, vice-president in leadership formation and former Vice-President for Catholic Health East writes: "As leadership has evolved and as management and governance roles have been filled increasingly by laypeople, the important role of leadership formation and leadership development has become even more critical."[72] He goes on to state:

> The implications of this 'second generation' phenomenon are quite profound, not only for those charged with the preparation and delivery of formal leadership formation and development programs, but for all who serve in leadership roles in Catholic health care.[73]

Intentional leadership formation in the mission and identity of Catholic health care must be priority, not just for leaders, but also for all who are involved in advancing its mission. Jeanne Buckeye and Michael Naughton, who have written extensively on leadership formation in Catholic health care, recognized that the setting and expectations have drastically changed:

> Today, Catholic health care and education function in environments more complex and challenging than any of the founders could have imagined in virtually every

---

72 Peter J. Giammalvo, "A 'Second Generation' of Ministry Leadership: How Do We Form Leaders Who Have Not Experienced Working Directly with Religious?" *Health Progress* (September-October 2005), 15-16.

73 Ibid., 16.

dimension: administrative; competitive; economic; legal; technical; social; workforce; and religious.[74]

Many business skills were needed and sought after in the hiring of Catholic health care leaders, but often, the Catholic mission and identity became secondary or was not even considered in the hiring process. There was a desire to provide solid leadership in regard to the market but not necessarily for the mission. Buckeye and Naughton again remark,

> Knowledge of the founding tradition, commitment to its religious vision – what became of these? It seems, at this stage, the distinctive mission was assumed but not cultivated. Legitimate concerns for leaders' character and administrative abilities were not matched by concern for their knowledge of the faith and traditions that had animated their founders. New leaders were selected with an almost naïve hope that (they) could pick up the Catholic vision as they worked.[75]

The expectation that Catholic health care leaders would be able to "pick up" what the founding sisters began in living the mission of Catholic health care, as a mission of the Church, was not always realized. Buckeye and Naughton name the problem today: "Thus came mission drift, an unprecedented movement away from the core purpose and vision of the organization, a movement powered by incremental and subtle changes arising from a series of decisions over time."[76] "Mission drift" continues

---

74 Buckeye and Naughton, *The Importance of Leadership Formation*, 38.

75 Ibid., 39.

76 Ibid., 39.

to affect the Catholic identity of the hospital and has brought about moral compromise on the teachings of the Church and the mission that was once guided by the religious.

Mergers of Catholic and Secular Health Care Institutions

Along with mission drift, leaders ill-formed in the mission of Catholic health care had to manage Catholic health care systems in a difficult market and learn how to partner with other health care systems. The *Ethical and Religious Directives* speak directly to this point.

In ever-increasing ways, Catholic health care providers have become involved with other health care organizations and providers. For instance, many Catholic health care systems and institutions share in the joint purchase of technology and services with other local facilities or physicians' groups. Another phenomenon is the growing number of Catholic health care systems and institutions joining or co-sponsoring integrated delivery networks or managed care organizations in order to contract with insurers and other health care payers.[77]

Because of the high costs of medicine, medical treatments, insurance, and a host of other factors, religious-based hospitals found it fiscally challenging to purchase state-of-the art equipment and electronic charting systems and to pay top dollar for expert physicians. To have market share or to stay competitive, Catholic hospitals often merged with other Christian or secular hospitals. John Gallagher, in his excellent article on this topic, writes:

The litmus test for Catholic health care organizations

---

77 *Ethical and Religious Directives,* Part Six "Forming New Partnerships with Health Care Organizations and Providers," 29.

43

is that a partnership cannot involve the Catholic organization in cooperating with objective moral evils, such as those procedures inconsistent with the Ethical and Religious Directives for Catholic Health Care Services, including direct sterilization, abortion, in vitro fertilization, inappropriate stem cell research, physician assisted suicide, and euthanasia.[78]

Although the decision to merge seemed to make sense to those in hospital leadership, due diligence from a moral and mission perspective was sometimes overlooked. The results were a weakening of the Catholic identity, inattentiveness to formation programs for merged leaders, and the provision of immoral services.

The challenges to the Catholic mission in health care have continued to increase. For example, external organizations hostile to the Catholic Church have lobbied against the mergers of non-Catholic facilities with Catholic systems so as to prevent the perceived loss of contraceptive services.[79] Government regulators have at times prohibited the sale of a non-Catholic facility to

---

78 John A. Gallagher, "Discerning the Future of the American Catholic Health Care Ministry." *The National Catholic Bioethics Quarterly*, Vol 13, Issue 2, (Summer 2013), 264. This is an excellent scholarly piece that describes the history of American medicine that led up to and contributed to many immoral mergers between Catholic and secular hospitals.

79 Takahashi, Joelle, Abigail Cher, Jeanelle Sheeder, Stephanie Teal and Maryam Guiahi. "Disclosure of Religious Identity and Health Care Practices on Catholic Hospital Websites." *Journal of the American Medical Association* (March 19, 2019), Vol. 321, Number 11. In this research letter, it is interesting to note that many Catholic hospitals fail to clearly identify themselves as Catholic hospitals, which the authors state, is deliberate to prevent certain health care procedures, especially reproductive procedures, from being offered to patients who came to them without this knowledge.

a Catholic facility because of public outcry over reduction in reproductive rights.[80] With a lack of formation in ERD and the Church's medical–moral teachings, Catholic identity has been compromised.

One such case is Mercy Hospital in Redding, California. It belonged to Dignity Health Care, part of a group of 29 hospitals, some bound by the ERD's and some not. The case revolved around sterilization procedures, something prohibited by number 53 of the ERD.[81] With a possible lawsuit being filed by the ACLU, "the (Catholic) hospital in Redding reversed its normal policy."[82] This "normal" way of behaving and acting in a Catholic hospital goes to the core of who we are as promoters and protectors of human life, especially at its earliest stage. This is not the only case where such challenges have happened. Because of lawsuit threats, public opinion and public pressures, many Catholic hospitals have found it difficult to remain faithful to the Church's teachings and its mission from Christ.

Lisa Gilden, general counsel for CHA, wrote of CHA's hope to provide other juridical structures that could be implemented with the current climate of mergers between Catholic and non-Catholic health systems. She writes:

> Currently, there are 41 Catholic hospitals in the United States that belong to other-than-Catholic

---

80 Nelson, *Diagnosis Critical*, 88-89. Nelson provides an excellent overview of a number of mergers, affiliations, and sales and gives the reasons why many Catholic hospitals moved in this direction.

81 *Ethical and Religious Directives*, 24.

82 James V. Schall, "Will Catholic Hospitals be the Next Target?" *Crisis*, September 2, 2015. https://www.crisismagazine.com/2015/will-catholic-hospitals-be-the-next-target (accessed on January 5, 2018).

systems. Of these, 22 are no longer sponsored by a religious congregation or public juridic person, but instead remain Catholic as a result of an agreement between the secular buyer and the applicable diocesan bishop.[83]

Mergers are becoming more common as systems become larger and acquire more of the market share and influence in buying power. The question that needs to be asked among Catholic health care sponsors and leaders, along with appropriate Church officials, is whether mergers, especially with non-Catholic facilities, will sustain Catholic health care as a ministry of the Church or cause the mission to be compromised because of public perception, scandal, or lack of due diligence. Gilden again writes:

> In some instances, Catholic systems and their sponsors have had to make the difficult decision to sell some or all of their hospitals. The preference would be to transfer the hospital to another Catholic sponsor and health system, but sometimes-financial circumstances, geographic location, market conditions or other factors make a match with an existing Catholic system unfeasible.[84]

---

83 Lisa Gilden, "Exploring Legal Models to Preserve Catholicity," *Health Progress* (May-June 2017), 35. The issue of mergers and the responsibility of sponsors, boards, and other procedures is addressed clearly in Part VI of the *Ethical and Religious Directives for Catholic Health Care Services*. See also the document from the Congregation for the Doctrine of the Faith, *Some Principles for Collaboration with non-Catholic Entities in the Provision of Healthcare Services* (February 17, 2014)

84 Ibid., 35.

As she notes, many of these decisions are extremely difficult to make and the resulting mergers have occasioned more harm to the mission than benefit. It is only with proper due diligence, process, formation, faith, and timely planning that mergers can be entered into so as to ensure the continued spiritual mission of Catholic health care and to sustain the hospital.

The *National Catholic Reporter* published an article on the moral compromises that mergers have often precipitated. Many Catholic hospital systems merged their formation programs with other non-Catholic hospitals they purchased, which led to compromising Catholic identity. They write:

> But although the nonprofit organizations operate as ministries of the Catholic Church, with a deep commitment to heal the sick and serve the poor, they are also businesses with a real need for funding to hire well-trained staff, buy new equipment and survive. Sometimes this means they have to form alliances with non-Catholic organizations, meld together missions and agree to compromise.[85]

Partnering with non-Catholic providers brings with it many challenges, one of which is its inattentiveness to following the original charism of the religious congregation. M. Therese Lysaught, a Catholic professor of bioethics and health policy, addresses this issue.

> Before moving forward, Catholic health care must analyze the moral dimensions of Catholic participation in clinically integrated networks, especially in light

---

85 Alice Popovici, "Shift to Laity Sparks Formation Needs." *National Catholic Reporter* (February 21, 2012).

of the fact that the United States Conference of Catholic Bishops has long recognized the necessity and value of forming new partnerships with health care organizations and providers. Yet all partnerships raise questions about the potential for issues of moral cooperation and scandal.[86]

Yet even with these disappointing situations, there have been successful mergers where the Catholic identity not only has been preserved but also enhanced and strengthened within the facility, its members, and in the community. The ERDs speak to this positive outcome: "On the other hand, new partnerships can be viewed as opportunities for Catholic health care institutions and services to witness to their religious and ethical commitments and so influence the healing profession."[87]

Conclusion

The moral and legal challenges to Catholic health care are immense. John Mudd underscores this thought, "To lose the voice, influence and care of Catholic hospitals and universities

---

86 M. Therese Lysaught, "Clinically Integrated Networks: A Cooperation Analysis." White Paper. Given to leaders at Trinity Health in 2013. https://www.chausa.org/publications/health-care-ethics-usa/archives/issues/fall-2015/clinically-integrated-networks-a-cooperation-analysis (accessed October 16, 2017).

87 *Ethical and Religious Directives*, 29. See also an article by *Modern Healthcare* in which they report that as Catholic systems have grown in acquiring more hospitals, there has been a sharp decrease in abortions, which is another positive outcome in the Church's continued care for the poor. http://www.modernhealthcare.com/article/20170914/NEWS/170919931 (accessed October 23, 2017). See the excellent article "As Catholic systems grow by acquiring other hospitals, abortions plummet" by Steven Ross Johnson in *Modern Healthcare* (September 14, 2017).

in our culture would be tragic. To reinforce these institutions as both Catholic and excellent is the challenge facing their sponsoring congregations and those in leadership positions."[88] Yet the mission of Catholic health care as a service to the poor, the vulnerable, the underinsured, and those without a community of faith is essential and must be secured so as to continue the saving ministry of Jesus. As Pope Francis has regularly remarked in regard to the mission of the Church that, "The Church must be like a field hospital that cleans and heals wounds."[89] Although Pope Francis may be referring to the Church's responsibility to heal the spiritual, emotional, and psychological wounds of God's people in the world, the analogy to a field hospital has undertones that can be met by those involved in Catholic health care. Gilden agrees that the mission of Catholic health care must continue.

> Maintaining a community's Catholic hospital allows it to continue to serve as a witness to Jesus' mission of love and healing. As both an employer and provider, Catholic hospitals answer God's call to foster healing, act with compassion and promote wellness for all persons and communities, with special attention to those who are poor, underserved, and most vulnerable.[90]

Saint John Paul II also saw these difficulties of our modern time when he wrote,

---

88 Mudd, 25.

89 Rome Reports, May 2, 2015. http://www.romereports.com/en/2015/02/05/pope-francis-homily-the-church-should-be-like-a-field-hospital/ (accessed October 23, 2017).

90 Gilden, 39.

Yet, there remains much we still must do if we are to ensure that the health care ministry is to remain 'one of the most vital apostolates of the ecclesial community and one of the most significant services which Christianity offers to society in the name of Jesus Christ.'[91]

Pellegrino and Thomasma sum up this chapter when speaking of health care reform: "The whole community, Christian and non-Christian, must ensure that fiscal exigency will not drive Catholic hospitals into either moral compromise or bankruptcy."[92] Mindful of the challenges of decreased leadership in Catholic health care ministry, the lack of theologically sound formation programs, and compromises that can come with mergers and the ever present challenges in the health care market, we look to Jesus who teaches us how to respond to those in need through the apostolate and mission of Catholic health care.

---

91 John Paul II, "Address to the Catholic Health Association," *L'Osservatore Romano* (September 21, 1987): 19.

92 Edmund D. Pellegrino and David C. Thomasma, "Charity in Action: Compassion and Caring." *The Christian Virtues in Medical Practice* (Washington, D.C.: Georgetown University Press, 1996), 91.

CHAPTER 3

The New Evangelization and the Call to Mission in Catholic Health Care

The early apostles, called by Jesus into the service of love and charity, called other followers of Jesus into that same service. These future disciples were missioned to serve Christ in the world, not always as ordained presbyters or leaders in the Church, but as baptized believers who shared the very life of Jesus.

In the current era of Catholic health care, we must return to and embrace the role of each baptized believer as a conduit of the healing mission of Christ through his or her own individual gifts, which are given by God for the building up of the Church. The consecrated religious, formed intentionally in the life and ministry of Jesus, completely gave of themselves in order to heal by loving others like Christ. The early religious in health care were first inspired by their own baptism to bring Christ's healing love to those in need. Thus, being incorporated into the very life of Jesus and strengthened by the embrace of the Evangelical Counsels (poverty, chastity and obedience that they vow to live by within their particular Community), the early religious fulfilled the needs of the Church as called forth by bishops and priest, as well as by their superiors.

In the early chapters, I referenced many scriptural texts that illuminated Jesus' healing love in his ministry of making the Kingdom of God present to the world. The apostles continued that healing love that Jesus first offered to them. One such apostle was St. Paul, a Pharisee and a member of the Jewish religious leadership whose role was to study the Laws of Israel and interpret them for the people.

The Call to Ministry in Ephesians 4:11-16

St. Paul was a devout Jew, committed to God and the Law of the Old Testament. St. Paul was so devout that he persecuted the early Christians, thinking he was being faithful to the will of God. The Acts of the Apostles (9:3-6) describes St. Paul's misguided attempts at following God:

> On his journey, as he was nearing Damascus, a light from the sky suddenly flashed around him. He fell to the ground and heard a voice saying to him, 'Saul, Saul, why are you persecuting me?' He said, 'Who are you, sir?' The reply came, 'I am Jesus, whom you are persecuting. Now get up and go into the city and you will be told what you must do."

Jesus said that St. Paul's persecution of the Christians was a direct attack upon him.[93]

St. Paul's conversion brought about a complete change of heart (*metanoia*), however, and he became a passionate follower of Jesus. Jesus was calling Paul into a personal relationship of love and service through his preaching of the Gospel. Following his conversion, St. Paul was sent to the known world as a light to the Gentiles (Acts 13:47 and 26:23). I would argue that this

---

93 Matthew 25:35-36 makes clear the response that Jesus asks us to make in his service. As often as we seek to meet the corporal and spiritual needs of others, we are fulfilling the healing will of Christ, "As often as you did it to the least of my brothers, you did it to me."

same call or mission is foundational to Jesus' disciples today, especially in the Church's mission of health care.

St. Paul's inspired vocation was to bring the saving message of Jesus to all people, Jew and Gentile alike.[94] One work of St. Paul that is seminal to our grasp of the ministry of Catholic health care is his letter to the Ephesians, particularly 4:11-16. The *Letter to the Ephesians,* (found in the New Testament of the Bible), is assumed by most as a Pauline corpus written later in his life, possibly while in prison in Rome.[95] Others posit that it was a pseudo-Pauline letter because of its difference in syntax and vocabulary as well as its form and structure.[96] For our purposes, we will recognize that the letter to the Ephesians was written by St. Paul to a number of communities around Ephesus in present day Turkey. There are many themes within the Letter, but the theme I wish to focus on is St. Paul's insight on the gifts of God given for ministry. These gifts, enumerated by St. Paul, can be used in health care ministry. One might immediately think of the gifts of the Holy Spirit, such as Wisdom, Understanding Counsel etc, and those seven fold gifts. Here I wish to refer to the gifts referenced by St. Paul in his letter to the Ephesians as gifts for leadership and evangelization. All the gifts of God are intended to build up the Church in the body of Christ. Health care is no exception.

St. Paul writes in Ephesians 4:11-16 that the gifts of the Holy

---

94 The scriptures speak of Paul's call by Jesus and Paul's understanding of this call. It can be found in Acts 26:19-23, 1 Corinthians 9:19-23, 2 Corinthians 10:16-17, and Galatians 1:11-17. Paul also makes reference to his call in other passages in his thirteen letters in the New Testament.

95 John Muddiman, *The Epistle to the Ephesians: Black's New Testament Commentaries* (New York, NY: Continuum, 2001), 2.

96 Ibid., 3-11.

Spirit are given to apostles, preachers, pastors, and teachers for the purpose of building up the body of Christ. The Holy Spirit bestowed individual gifts or charisms so that the call to sanctify the world for Christ would continue long after the death of the apostles. *Lumen Gentium* speaks unmistakably to this need:

> "Guiding the Church in the way of all truth (cf. Jn 16:13) and unifying her in communion and in the works of ministry, he bestows upon her varied hierarchical and charismatic gifts, and in this way directs her; and he adorns her with his fruits (cf. Eph 4:11-12; 1 Cor. 12:4; Gal. 5:22)."[97]

The Congregation for the Doctrine of the Faith, in its document on the "Relationship Between Hierarchical and Charismatic Gifts in the Life and the Mission of the Church," states that these gifts of the Holy Spirit must have at their core charity and the desire to build up the Church. "These authorities should, to this end, bear in mind the unforeseeable nature of the charisms inspired by the Holy Spirit and evaluate them according to the rule of faith with the intention of building up the Church."[98]

When we think about the Holy Spirit being bestowed upon the Church, we often think of the Feast of Pentecost where the Holy Spirit came upon the apostles to give them courage to preach the Gospel message and to evangelize the

---

97 *Lumen Gentium*, 4.

98 Congregation for the Doctrine of the Faith, *Iuvenescit Ecclesiae, Relationship Between Hierarchical and Charismatic Gifts in the Life and the Mission of the Church*, (May 15, 2016), 17. http://www.vatican.va/roman_curia/congregations/cfaith/documents/rc_con_cfaith_doc_20160516_iuvenescit-ecclesia_en.html (accessed on December 18, 2017).

known world in name of Christ (see Acts 2). The Holy Spirit is also given to people today in a profound way in the Sacrament of Baptism and Confirmation. Anyone who accepts the Holy Spirit, in the name of Jesus, is baptized in that Spirit. It is the Holy Spirit who missions each follower to preach and teach in the name of Christ. St. Paul is a perfect example of this gift!

There are some Christians who have received the sacramental gift of baptism but who have not fully embraced the Spirit's gift for ministry. Francis Sullivan sees the "baptism of the spirit" in all who call upon the Holy Spirit for help and guidance and truly believe that baptism in the Spirit is distinct from the sacramental experience of baptism. Ralph Martin, viewing the issue differently, sees sacramental graces coming from the gift of baptism itself. Martin, quoting Francis Sullivan on the Holy Spirit says this, "He (Sullivan) proposes that baptism in the Spirit may perhaps more appropriately be seen as a distinct sending of the Spirit, apart from Christian initiation, to equip the recipient for a special service or for an important step forward in life with Christ."99 When a person calls upon the Holy Spirit and is filled with that Spirit to evangelize in Jesus' name, he/she can accomplish amazing things. What propelled Jesus forward in his mission was love. It was to bring the love of the Father through forgiveness of sin to every relationship. This type of love, lived and proclaimed by Jesus, should be the pledge of all those who heal and teach in Jesus' name. It is this love through the Holy Spirit that we are equipped with when those in Catholic health care minister

---

99 Ralph Martin, "A New Pentecost? Catholic Theology and 'Baptism in the Spirit,'" *Logos* 14:3 (Summer, 2011), 24. Martin proposes that not only are we given the gift of the Spirit at the Sacrament of Initiation, but we are also given the gift of the Holy Spirit for a special work, especially in the life of the Church.

in God's name. Avery Cardinal Dulles, an eminent Church scholar, confirms this: "Love transforms the heralds into living witnesses who testify not only by their words but by all that they do and are."100 Catholic health care leaders will be aided and sustained by the Holy Spirit when they embrace these gifts given to them by the Church.

In regard to the gifts given as outlined in Ephesians, Peter Williamson says: "God gives people to serve the Church, and he equips them with the natural and supernatural abilities necessary to fulfill these roles."[101]

Leaders in Catholic health care, especially those baptized in Christ, have the inner life of the Trinity dwelling within them. With that indwelling, these roles given by the Spirit as evangelizers, especially in witnessing to one's faith in Christ and sharing that faith with staff and patients within the Catholic health care setting, will allow that gift to build up the Church in love. The role of apostles belongs to Bishops as successors of the Apostles. Bishops teach, preach and govern in the name of the Church and their role in assuring that health care is a ministry of the Church and finds ratification in the words of St. Paul to the Ephesians. As Bishops preach and teach, which is the particular role of an evangelizer, those baptized in Christ, according to the teaching of the Second Vatican Council, also share in this role in sanctifying the world. Sanctifying the world in Catholic health care as baptized disciples of Jesus emboldens the believers and thus enables these gifts to be lived

---

100 Avery Dulles, "The Charism of the New Evangelizer," *Retrieving Charisms for the Twenty-First Century*, Doris Donnelly, ed. (Collegeville, MN: The Liturgical Press, 1999), 43.

101 Peter S. Williamson, *Ephesians* (Grand Rapids, MI: Baker Academic, 2009), 116. See also Peter T. O'Brien in his helpful commentary on Ephesians, pages 2-4.

and carried out so that Catholic health care can be a ministry of the whole Church.

The role of apostles and prophets were foundational in the life of the Church because they were the direct link to God's saving message and work in the Old Testament and the New Testament. Evangelists, as St. Paul mentions, are those "who would be engaged in the preaching of the gospel."[102] In 2 Timothy 4:5 St. Paul tells Timothy, "as for you, always be steady, endure suffering, do the work of an evangelist, fulfill your ministry." In Acts 21:8, Paul says he "entered the house of Philip the evangelist…" Although little is known about the particular role of evangelist in the early Church, Peter Williamson remarks, "It seems that evangelists, like apostles, announced the good news of salvation in Jesus and summoned their hearers to conversion."[103]

Pastors and teachers are mentioned last in St. Paul's listing of roles for the building up of the Church. Pastors and teachers embraced a very important role in encouraging their hearers to respond to their message by living according to the commandments and the teachings of the Church as a household community and therefore helping fellow disciples to live their lives in union with Christ.

Leadership in the Church is linked with service, as Jesus modeled true service for his apostles when he washed their feet (John 13:1-17). St. Paul, following Jesus' mandate to serve others, enumerates these particular roles found in Ephesians 4:11-16. Verse 11 in particular, challenges each Christian believer to become equipped (*kakartismos*); other translations define this word as perfected for the ministry they

---

102 Ibid., 299.

103 Williamson, *Ephesians*, 117.

have been called to offer. Williamson, following up on verse 11 of Ephesians, states that these roles have been established "to equip the holy ones for the work of ministry, in other words, to prepare the members of the Church, particularly the laity, to accomplish all that ministry entails."104

In each Christian community that Paul evangelized, there was a need to form (equip) leaders to encourage (Ephesians 6:22, 1 Thessalonians 5:11), exhort (1 Thessalonians 4:10, 1 Timothy 5:1), and teach (Romans 2:21, 1 Corinthians 4:17, Titus 2:1) in the name of Jesus. Leadership was entrusted to spirit-filled people as pastors and teachers, but many other roles of service were also fulfilled by the community's embracing St. Paul's preaching. St. Paul preached leadership in the Church, but a leadership based on service in the name of Christ (Romans 12:7, 1 Corinthians 12:5, Ephesians 6:7). St. John Chrysostom, commenting on these verses from Ephesians writes, "Perceive ye the value and dignity of the office? Each one edifies, each one perfects, each one ministers."105 The holy ones (*hagios*)106 (Ephesians 4:12) the baptized followers of Christ who have heard the message, believed it (Ephesians 1:13), and carried out the work, under the inspiration of the Holy Spirit, of building

---

104 Williamson, *Ephesians*, 117.

105 John Chrysostom, *Commentary on the Epistle to the Galatians and Homilies on the Epistle to the Ephesians: Homily XI, translated by Members of the English Church: A Library of Fathers of the Holy Catholic Church, Anterior Division of the East and West* (London, UK: Oxford, 1845), 223-224.

106 Blue Letter Bible references *hagios* as holy 161 times, saints 61 times, and Holy One 4 times. It is important to recognize the call to be holy, set-apart, God-like if we are going to minister in the name of Christ. https://www.blueletterbible.org/lang/lexicon/lexicon. cfm?Strongs=G40&t=RSV (accessed on December 3, 2017)

up the body of Christ (Ephesians 4:12, 16). These gifts were and are given to all members of the Church, each to his or her own ability, so that together, as a community, each may build up the body of Christ in healing and love.

Williamson brings to a close these profound verses of Ephesians 4:11-16:

> To summarize, Paul is saying that the goal of the diverse gifts Jesus gives the Church is ministry that leads to Christ-like maturity in the body as a whole and in its individual members. This maturity is characterized by a unity in doctrine, relationships with Christ himself, and stable adherence to the truth. It involves sincere conduct and love and requires that each member of the body of Christ fulfill his or her role of service.[107]

In Ephesians 4:11, St. Paul emphasized that spiritual gifts were given for ministry and to equip the holy ones (v 12) for the particular work God has entrusted to them.

In conclusion, St. Paul's preaching, particularly in Ephesians 4:11-16, can assist us in equipping and preparing the people of God, the lay baptized men and women, for the work of ministry, so that God's work of healing in our Catholic health care facilities will continually be carried out. Ephesians can inform, guide, and equip Catholic health care leaders in this great ministry of love in the name of Christ and as a mission of the Church.

Equipping Catholic Health Care Leaders

Evangelization is the making of Jesus as Lord and Savior known

---

107 Williamson, *Ephesians*, 123.

to the whole world, and it is centered in Jesus Christ, the Son of God who was sent by the Father to offer salvation to mankind. Evangelization is the proclamation of the saving name of Jesus Christ who died so that all people could have life. This proclamation is directed to all the nations. The Pontifical Council for Health Care Workers in its statement on evangelization writes, "The New Evangelization must be ever aware of the Paschal Mystery of the death and resurrection of Jesus Christ."[108] Evangelization was the goal of the apostles and disciples of Jesus, and it is still the Church's goal, especially in the field of health care.

The Holy Spirit has been active in the life of the Church since Pentecost (see Acts 2). It was the Holy Spirit who inspired St. John XXIII to call for the 21st Ecumenical Council (better known as the Second Vatican Council) so that the bishops could discuss how the Church should continue to preach the Gospel of Jesus Christ in the modern world.[109] More than sixteen documents were produced from the prayer and work of the bishops and many scholars. Avery Dulles, who was present at the Council, recognized the essential role of evangelization as called forth by documents of the Second Vatican Council:

> The teaching of Vatican II is fundamental to the concept of the "new evangelization." The Council describes evangelization as a task of the whole Church, which shares in the prophetic office of Christ the Lord (*LG* §12; cf. *Dignitatis Humanae* § 13). "Since the

---

108 The Pontifical Council for Health Care Workers, *Pastoral Care in Health and the New Evangelization for the Transmission of the Faith*, 6.

109 John XXIII felt a sudden "inspiration" to call for a Council of the world's bishops and to seek the guidance of the Holy Spirit. He also established the preparatory commission on Pentecost in 1959 and on Pentecost a year later began to synthesize the material for the Council.

whole Church is missionary, and since the work of evangelization is a basic duty of the People of God, this sacred Synod summons all to a deep interior renewal" (*Ad Gentes* § 35).[110]

Of all the Vatican II documents, *Lumen Gentium* (A Light to the Nations) is often recognized as the foundational one. In this Dogmatic Constitution on the Church, Jesus is described as the source of light and the center of all creation. Many of the other documents of the Second Vatican Council can be glimpsed within this document. *Lumen Gentium* shows the role of the Holy Spirit as the giver of all gifts and the one who inspires and makes effective the mission of salvation, especially when those called respond in faith.[111]

John W. O'Malley, commenting on *Lumen Gentium* in his work on the Second Vatican Council, summarizes the role of each baptized Christian to be a light in the world for Christ:

Christ, it insisted, calls every Christian to holiness and provides the grace and other means to accomplish it, regardless of one's state in life. Christians fulfill the call through love of God and neighbor in imitation of Christ, an imitation that takes on a rich variety of forms.[112]

Gaudium et Spes is another major Constitution of the documents of the Second Vatican Council (On the Church in the Modern World); it called the already baptized followers of Jesus into a deeper relationship with him through the Holy

---

110 Dulles, *The Charism of the New Evangelizer*, 38.

111 *Lumen Gentium*, 2 & 4.

112 John W. O'Malley, *What Happened at Vatican II* (Cambridge, MA: Harvard University Press, 2008), 174.

Spirit. Those baptized followers were called to share the Good News of salvation with those in the world who are without hope, purpose, or meaning.

Pope Saint Paul VI (1963-1978), as Pope of the post-conciliar Church, was instrumental in calling for a renewed spirit of evangelization. When he took the name of Paul, it was a foreshadowing of his desire to be a great missionary and evangelist like St. Paul. In 1975, Pope Paul VI wrote *Evangelii Nuntiandi* (Evangelization in the Modern World). *Evangelii Nuntiandi* describes not only the social evils of our time, but it teaches that it is only Jesus who can free us from all oppression, especially the oppression of sin.

> Evangelization will also always contain – as the foundation, center, and at the same time, summit of its dynamism- a clear proclamation that, in Jesus Christ, the Son of God made man, who died and rose from the dead, salvation is offered to all men, as a gift of God's grace and mercy.[113]

Saint John Paul II relied on Blessed Paul VI's definition of evangelization in *Evangelii Nuntiandi* and in many of his other writings. Pope Emeritus Benedict XVI and Pope Francis have also frequently quoted *Evangelii Nuntiandi* . Along with the guidance of the Second Vatican Council in preaching the message of Christ to the modern world, Pope Saint Paul VI proposed that it is the role of the whole Church to offer Jesus' saving love. In regard to the work of evangelization in the context of secularism, he stated the following:

As a result of the frequent situations of dechristianiza-

---

113 Paul VI, *Evangelii Nuntiandi*, 27.

tion in our day, [evangelization] also proves equally necessary for innumerable people who have been baptized but who live quite outside Christian life, for simple people who have a certain faith but an imperfect knowledge of the foundations of that faith, for intellectuals who feel the need to know Jesus Christ in a light different from the instruction they received as children, and for many others.[114]

Paul VI was addressing the need to re-evangelize all people in an increasingly secular culture with the truth of Jesus Christ.

Saint John Paul II also observed the secularization of the world and its ravaging effects upon faith and the family, a depersonalization of human life, and a weakening of faith, and he realized that what Pope Saint Paul VI had written about healing the world was precisely the focus he would continue in his pontificate. A statement by the United States Conference of Catholic Bishops (USCCB) summarizes this progression well.

While the need for a renewed evangelization of the baptized was first formally articulated by Pope Paul VI in *Evangelii Nuntiandi* and stems back to the calling of the Second Vatican Council, it was St. John Paul II who, in 1983, formally called this pastoral strategy the "new evangelization."[115]

Saint John Paul II first used the term *new evangelization*

---

114 Ibid., 52. Paul VI's document is a must read for those who want to renew the world for Christ. He identifies the great need of proclaiming as ever new and with new enthusiasm the saving message of Jesus.

115 United States Conference of Catholic Bishops, *Living as Missionary Disciples: A Resource for Evangelization* (Washington, D.C.: USCCB Publishing, 2017), 7.

early writings, especially in his address to the Latin ...merican Bishops in 1983. Evangelization is not new to the followers of Jesus, but it is new in its "ardor, methods and expression,"[116] the Pope said. John Paul II said that evangelization is to be directed to three groups: (1) those who have not heard the Gospel, (2) those who have a relationship with Jesus but need to be renewed and grow more deeply in that relationship, (3) those fallen away Catholics who are not living their sacramentalized life in Christ.[117] "He [John Paul II] clarified that the new evangelization is new, not in content but rather in its inner thrust; new in its methods that must correspond to the times; and new because it is necessary to proclaim the Gospel to those who have already heard it."[118]

With regard to Catholic health care and the new evangelization, the Pontifical Council for Health Care Workers defines the term this way:

> The new evangelization, therefore, does not necessarily require the invention of something new to be done, but rather, the promotion and strengthening in all

---

116 John Paul II, Opening Address to the Assembly of CELAM, Port-au-Prince, Haiti, March 9, 1983 (translation from *L'Osservatore Romano* English Edition 16/780, April 18, 1983, no. 9). Therese Lysaught provides a clear connection to the new evangelization in Catholic health care in her book *Caritas in Communion: Theological Foundations of Catholic Health Care* (St. Louis, MO: Catholic Health Association, 2014), 41-43.

117 John Paul II, *Redemptoris Missio*, (The Mission of the Redeemer), 7 December 1990. http://w2.vatican.va/content/john-paul-ii/en/encyclicals/documents/hf_jp-ii_enc_07121990_redemptoris-missio.html (accessed on December 12, 2017).

118 United States Conference of Catholic Bishops, *Disciples Called to Witness* (Washington, D.C.: USCCB Publishing, 2012), 6.

believers of a common and shared vision of reality which springs from faith, and which in its turn generates a [*sic*] 'new' way of thinking about human life and a new way of acting towards it in relation to everything that concerns it...[119]

The new evangelization is also new because the proclamation of the gospel is not just meant to be accomplished by priestly missionaries; the good news of Jesus' proclamation is meant to be proclaimed by all the baptized, including and most importantly, especially for our purposes, those leading the Church's apostolate in health care.

Even though the baptized followers of Christ have heard the message, they have not always responded to the message of Jesus. Some would say they have been sacramentalized with the sacraments but not evangelized with the saving message of Jesus. Pope Francis also challenged all the baptized to "move beyond a dull or mechanical way of living our faith, and instead open the doors of our hearts, our lives, our parishes, our movements or associations, going out in search of others so as to bring them the light and the joy of our faith in Christ."[120]

The Laity's Call to Ministry

The mission of Catholic health care as an apostolate of all members of the Church has been affirmed and strengthened in the modern era, especially in the writings of the documents of

---

119 The Pontifical Council for Health Care Workers, *Pastoral Care*, 41-42. John Paul II saw first-hand the de-Christianization that was occurring in Europe, especially in the political arena, and he wanted to reawaken, in particular, the faith of people in the traditionally Christian parts of Europe.

120 Pope Francis, *General Audience*, March 27, 2013.

the Second Vatican Council when the Council Fathers called the laity to participation and leadership in the mission of the Church. The Decree on the Laity states:

> To intensify the apostolic activity of the people of God, the most holy synod earnestly addresses itself to the laity, whose proper and indispensable role in the mission of the Church has already been dealt with in other documents. The apostolate of the laity derives from their Christian vocation and the Church can never be without it... Our own times require of the laity no less zeal: in fact, modern conditions demand that their apostolate be broadened and intensified.[121]

This demand for the laity's involvement in the apostolate of the Church, of which Catholic health care is a particular and important work of evangelization, is found in *Lumen Gentium*, which speaks of the role of the faithful in building up, healing, and sanctifying the Body of Christ.

> As all the members of the human body, though they are many, form one body, so also are the faithful in Christ. Also, in the building up of Christ's Body various members and functions have their part to play. There is only one Spirit who, according to His own richness and the needs of the ministries, gives His different gifts for the welfare of the Church.[122]

---

121 *Apostolicam Acousitatem*, 1. See also number 8 and 31 that speak well to this point.

122 *Lumen Gentium*, 7. *Lumen Gentium* 33-34 speaks clearly of the role the lay faithful who are baptized in Jesus' own death and resurrection can play in the mission of love in the world. See also *Gaudium et Spes* 11, 43-44, 52, and 62, which give encouragement to the laity to act in the mission of the Church, especially in Catholic health care.

The Pontifical Council for Health Care Workers confirms this vital role of caring for those in need:

> In wanting to take on 'The joys and the hopes, the griefs and the anxieties of the men of this age, especially those who are poor or in any afflicted', the Church today looks at the world of health, which is characterized by so many changes and problems, with the same compassion with which Jesus received the troubled and abandoned crowds of Galilee.[123]

With this strengthening of the religious roles of the laity within the Church, a newly recovered vision for the future has emerged: the mission and role of the laity and their call to sanctify the world and to participate in the new evangelization as called forth by the Church, especially in Catholic health care.

The challenges in Catholic health care, described earlier, are being met in many instances, especially in the increasing role and formation of the laity in leadership and in the mission and purpose of Catholic health care as enumerated by the Church's longstanding teaching from Jesus. Catholic health care has a new opportunity for the fulfillment of God's plan so that the mission of the laity in the world, called for by the Second Vatican Council, can be realized. Previously, the laity were defined in a negative light as those who were not ordained. The Second Vatican Council made every attempt to promote the rightful role of the lay faithful in building up and sanctifying the Church in the modern world. John W. O'Malley makes this point, "What, then, were, the most

---

123 Pontifical Council for Health Care Workers, *Pastoral Care in Health and the New Evangelization for the Transmission of the Faith*, 13.

important issues at the Council? The desire to recognize the dignity of lay men and women and to empower them to fulfill their vocation in the church was certainly among them."[124]

Who are the laity? The laity are the baptized Christians who seek the kingdom of God "by engaging in temporal affairs and directing them according to God's will. Living in the world, they are engaged in each and every work and business of the earth and in the ordinary circumstances of social and family life which constitute their very existence."[125] *Lumen Gentium* and *Gaudium et Spes* spoke directly to the important role the laity would be called upon to exercise in the future of the Church in the modern world.

Prior to the Second Vatican Council, there was an emphasis on the role of the ordained in ministering to the world in the name of the Church. With the Holy Spirit's guidance, the Council Fathers recognized and reaffirmed the role of the laity and how clergy and laity must work together to advance the Gospel of Jesus. Avery Cardinal Dulles wisely comments: "Christ continues to proclaim the Kingdom through the laity as well as through the ordained."[126]

Both clergy and laity are called to holiness in an equal manner and to share together in Christ's three-fold mission as priest, prophet, and king. St. Francis DeSales understood the individual call to holiness of each baptized member of the

---

124 O'Malley, 5. O'Malley goes on to comment that the decree dealing with the apostolate of the laity made it through the Council with relative ease because of the near universal agreement on the direction being taken.

125 *Lumen Gentium*, 31.

126 Avery Dulles, "The Charism of the New Evangelizer," in *Retrieving Charisms for the Twenty-First Century*, Doris Donnelly, ed. (Collegeville, MN: The Liturgical Press, 1999), 38

Church when we wrote his treatise, *Introduction to the Dev* *Life*. He foresaw that all members of the Church are called to holiness but each in his or her own way. Both clergy and laity are charged, entrusted, and missioned for seeking the holiness of all people in the world. *Gaudium et Spes* confirms this mission:

> Thus the Church, at once a visible association and a spiritual community, goes forth together with humanity and experiences the same earthly lot, which the world does. She serves as a leaven and as a kind of soul for human society as it is to be renewed in Christ and transformed into God's family. The role of the laity is the renewal of the temporal order by living the life of Christ fully and with authenticity.[127]

Ad Gentes, another document of the Second Vatican Council that fostered the role of the laity, says this: "Since the whole Church is missionary, and since the work of evangelization is a basic duty of the People of God, this sacred Synod summons all to a deep interior renewal."[128] The Second Vatican Council understood that assisting the Holy Spirit in bringing about holiness in the world for Christ was a responsibility of all the baptized. Edward Hahnenberg agrees: "The responsibility to

---

127 *Gaudium et Spes*, 40.

128 *Ad Gentes*, 35. The term "People of God" was of great importance in the section of *Lumen Gentium*; indeed, the entire section (nos. 9-17 & 18) was titled, "On the People of God." This same theme, to a lesser degree, is continued in *Gaudium et Spes*, in the Preamble, no. 3 and in Part One, no. 11. The term "people of God" describes biblical imagery often found in the Old Testament. Joseph Ratzinger, *Theological Highlights of Vatican II* (New York, NY: Paulist Press, 1966), writes, "By contrast, the new text returned wholeheartedly to the total biblical testimony about the Church. Here the idea of the 'body of Christ' is complemented with that of the 'People of God,'" 74.

transform the secular world according to the light of Christ does not belong to the laity alone. It is the responsibility of the whole Church."[129] Pope Francis echoes this same sentiment:

> In virtue of their baptism, all members of the People of God have become missionary disciples (cf. Mt 28:19). All the baptized, whatever their position in the Church or their level of instruction in the faith, are agents of evangelization, and it would be insufficient to envisage a plan of evangelization to be carried out by professionals while the rest of the faithful would simply be passive recipients. The new evangelization calls for personal involvement on the part of each of the baptized.[130]

Those who minister in the field of Catholic health care must live the saving mission of Jesus in their daily lives by caring for those in need and by proclaiming his saving love. We will now turn our attention to the healing mission of Catholic health care.

The Mission of Catholic Health Care as an Apostolate of the Laity

The mission of making Jesus known as Lord and Savior in the Church's health care ministry is paramount. As The Pontifical Council for Health Care Workers noted, "The Synod Fathers also pointed to the world of health as a 'specific' and 'proper'

---

129 Edward Hahnenberg, "Ordained and Lay Ministry: Restarting the Conversation," *Origins*, Vol. 35, No. 6 (June 23, 2005), 96. See his article on the role of clergy and laity, ministry and apostolate.

130 Pope Francis, *The Joy of the Gospel*, 91-92.

place for evangelization. On this subject they wrote: 'The Gospel also illumines the suffering brought about by disease. Christians must help the sick feel that the Church is near to persons with illness or disabilities.'"[131] Pope Francis has called us to serve the poor and those in need with greater intensity. He states, "When we read the Gospel we find a clear indication: not so much our friends and wealthy neighbors, but above all the poor and the sick, those who are usually despised and overlooked, 'those who cannot repay you' (Lk 14:14)."[132]

As the mission of Catholic health care in the United States continued to expand, there was a stark recognition, as we have pointed out, that the number of vowed religious would not be able to sustain the ministry of Catholic health care in the future. William Cox, president and CEO of the Alliance of Catholic Healthcare in California, describes the situation so deftly we find ourselves in today:

> For nearly 300 years, the Catholic mission in health care in the United States has been nurtured by thousands of religious sisters who founded and operated Catholic health care facilities and brought to them—in the words of the first president of the Catholic Health Association—"a spirit, a soul, an atmosphere and ideal of service... which they created and maintained and gave their lives' best efforts to foster." Today, those culture-bearers are largely absent from the administration of Catholic Health Care organizations and less available for their governance. Without the

---

131 The Pontifical Council for Health Care Workers, *Pastoral Care in Health and the New Evangelization for the Transmission of the Faith*, 5.

132 Pope Francis, *The Joy of the Gospel*, 42.

pervasive presence of the sisters, the question is, how will the culture of Catholic health care be sustained and transmitted to the next generation of Catholic Health Care leaders?[133]

The challenges outlined previously are being met with an increased formation process for the lay faithful in leadership in Catholic health care. From the comments addressed to sponsors and Catholic health care leaders cited previously came the agreement in California and across the United States that all "participants overwhelmingly identified an opportunity for collective action: 'Developing and implementing a leadership program for formation with common foundations.'"[134] Along with the decrease in religious leadership there began to develop a recognition that the formation of the next generation of leaders, especially the laity, would be needed and expected if Catholic health care was to be an effective instrument of the new evangelization.

The first draft of the ERD's in the early 1970's recognized that the laity would have to embrace leadership in Catholic health care: "The laity's participation and leadership in the health care ministry, through new forms of sponsorship and governance of institutional Catholic health care, are essential for the Church to continue her ministry of healing and compassion."[135] Andre Delbecq, Jack Mudd, and Celeste Mueller also capture the urgent necessity of formation for

---

133 William Cox, quoted in Lawrence J. O'Connell and John Shea, *Tradition on the Move: Leadership Formation in Catholic Health Care*, editors. (Sacramento, CA: MLC Press, 2013), 1-2.

134 Ibid., 2.

135 *Ethical and Religious Directives*, 4.

Catholic health care leaders and other Catholic institutions in an excellent article titled "Formation of Organizational Leaders for Catholic Mission and Identity." They sum up this urgent concern this way: "By contrast, the religious/theological education of leaders (if there has been any formal training) is often truncated at a less advanced level."[136] As the three authors recognize, the investment in resources for formation of lay leaders has taken place in earnest beginning in early 1990's with many larger hospital systems. "With greater discretionary resources Catholic healthcare, particularly the larger systems, have invested extensively in Mission and Identity formation..."[137] This is illustrated in several examples: the Ministry Leadership Formation Program (MLFP) of OSF Healthcare in Peoria, Illinois; the Ministry Leadership Center (established in 2002 by six Catholic health care systems with more than 700 leaders);[138] and the Catholic Health Association survey in 2010 on "Gauging Formation Effectiveness."

With recognition that formation is needed for Catholic health care leaders, the question then becomes, What kind of leadership? Is formation in business tactics, market share, and competitive edges, as was experimented with in Catholic health care in the late 1960s and 1970s, enough? No. Formation must include (1) knowledge and an embrace of Jesus Christ,

---

136 Andre L. Delbecq, Jack Mudd, and Celeste Mueller, "Formation of Organizational Leaders for Catholic Mission and Identity," *Journal of Jesuit Business Education* (Summer, 2012), 58.

137 Ibid., 58.

138 O'Connell and Shea, *Tradition on the Move*, XI. Their work is an excellent summary, from beginning to end, of how the realization of a need turned into an organization, in union with the local Bishop, dedicated solely to the formation of Catholic health care in the West.

(2) knowledge of the Catholic identity, and (3) secular skills. Delbecq and his co-authors put it this way:

> If we do not have a religiously grounded, theologically articulated understanding of who we are (within Catholic institutions) we will lose our way in this complex context. At the same time if we specify our identity but we cannot meet the standards of a rational, secular, pluralistic world, then our identity will not be effective.[139]

Archbishop Charles Chaput emphasized the importance of the mission and ministry of the Church in his address to Catholic medical personnel in 2010. He said that health care workers who are willing to stand up for their convictions as Catholics must see the teachings of Jesus in health care as a ministry.

> If you are one of the many in Catholic health care who see the Church and her teachings as the ministry of Jesus himself and seek God in your vocation and see the face of Christ in the suffering persons you help, then you are what the soul of the Catholic health care vocation has always been about.[140]

Sr. Teresa Stanley echoes this same thought as Archbishop Chaput:

> In whatever form they take, these programs teach leaders about the institution and Catholic health care

---

139 Delbecq, *Formation of Organizational Leaders*, 58.

140 Charles Chaput, "The Future of the Catholic Health Care Vocation," *Origins* 39, No. 40 (March 18, 2010), 657.

as a ministry rooted in Jesus. They also communicate the leaders' role in helping other associates connect the dots between their daily work and the ministry.[141]

Conclusion

The laity whose proper role it is to continue Jesus' saving ministry in the world must carry on Jesus' ministry in Catholic health care with intensity and determination. But, what does this intentional formation look like? Formation must include a well-developed and structured process whereby Jesus' healing love is seen first-hand in the care of the sick. It must include a passionate love to proclaim God's kingdom. If the Church can help form leaders so that they become true believers in Jesus who also desire to continue the rich apostolate of Catholic health care in the world as called forth by the Second Vatican Council, then the apostolate of Catholic health care will be sustained and be an effective means of evangelization in the world.

---

141 Stanley, *Can the Ministry Collaborate*, 13.

CHAPTER 4
The Future of Catholic Health Care Ministry

Within the discussion of Catholic health care, one often observes words such as reshaping, formation, leadership, transmission, renewing, and strengthening. These words, expressed by many in the forefront of Catholic health care, point to the pressing need to renew Catholic health care as a mission of the Church in the world. Jeanne Buckeye echoes this urgent need: "New attention is being paid to understanding Catholic mission and its theological roots, to the idea of Catholicity and to the ecclesial dimensions of a Catholic institution."[142] The revitalization and strengthening of Catholic health care in the United States must include a renewed emphasis on the formation of health care leaders through well-defined programs that aim to support and nourish the baptismal dignity of the laity now involved in Catholic health care. The Pontifical Council for Health Care Workers writes of the imperative renewal in formation:

> Formation offers to the Church an opportunity to be present in the health-care world to connect man to the transcendent when faced with the instability that is produced in him by illness; to proclaim and bear witness to the religious values of life, taken on as an end to which to consecrate one's existence; and to educate people in mutual compassion and mutual

---

142 Jeanne Buckeye, *The Importance of Leadership Formation*, 39.

solidarity at the beginning of an authentic journey of communion.[143]

The document goes on to clarify what formation must consist of:

Only by becoming aware of the centrality of man in his condition of weakness and frailty will a hospital remain 'a place in which the relationship of treatment is not a profession but a mission; where the charity of the Good Samaritan is the first seat of learning and the face of suffering man is Christ's own Face: "you did it to me"' (Mt 25:40).[144]

Therefore, leadership formation programs must include sustained spiritual development over a period of time, with goals and objectives in core competencies. Formation must also include opportunities for leaders to embrace Jesus' active healing in the world through the mission of Catholic health care as an essential part of what they do. Fr. Gerald Arbuckle in an insightful piece summarizes:

The lesson for today's leaders of Catholic health care is this: They need to be proactive in fostering prophetic cultures now. At stake is the very survival and growth of Catholic health care ministries. Ensuring survival and growth requires that people with prophetic gifts be identified and invited to lead our ministries.[145]

---

143 The Pontifical Council for Health Care Workers, *Pastoral Care in Health and the New Evangelization for the Transmission of the Faith*, 38.

144 Ibid., 38.

145 Arbuckle, *Maintaining Prophetic Cultures*, 24. I believe that Ar-

The Urgency of
Ministry Leadership Formation

At the center of formation and the ministry of evangelization is Jesus. Arbuckle makes the same point, "Leaders of contemporary and future health care ministries are called to build healing cultures of hope that are centered on Jesus Christ and his mission, not on themselves."[146] It is not enough to know Jesus as a popular figure in time, but Jesus must be known personally as Lord and Savior. Pope Benedict XVI addressed this same concern in *Jesus of Nazareth*, where he wrote: "This is a dramatic situation for faith, because its point of reference is being placed in doubt: Intimate friendship with Jesus, on which everything depends, is in danger of clutching at thin air."[147] A personal relationship with Jesus, which Catholic health care leaders and all baptized Christians are called to embrace, will only happen when leaders are provided the time and given the expectation of getting to know Jesus as Savior and Lord. Pope Benedict continued this same emphasis on Jesus in his encyclical *Deus Caritas Est*. Daniel Sulmasy, a physician and

---

buckle clearly identifies the threats to the mission of Catholic health care in this article. Raising up prophetic, holy, and spirit-led leaders renews the mission of Catholic health care because leaders will be challenged to address the full Catholic identity of this apostolate.

146 Ibid., 21.

147 Pope Benedict, *Jesus of Nazareth* (New York, NY: Doubleday, 2007), vii. Pope Benedict XVI addresses the topic that Jesus was and is a real person who came to reveal the love of God and to save us by his death on the cross. His book is an excellent answer and resource for those yearning to be leaders in Catholic health care who truly need to know and experience who Jesus is. See M. Therese Lysaught's work on the foundation of love in Catholic health care in her book *Caritas in Communion* (St. Louis, MO: Catholic Health Association, 2014), especially page 121.

Franciscan friar, who speaks on the importance of the love of Christ as the heart of Catholic health care writes, quoting Pope Benedict,

> Pope Benedict XVI begins by reminding us that the religion we profess, which is the foundation and the rationale for Catholic health care, is not an ideology. Nor is it a philosophy of life or even a moral code. It is, in the first instance, an encounter—an encounter with a Person—an encounter that changes everything.[148]

Archbishop Joseph F. Naumann, speaking to those in attendance at a White Mass, a Mass recognizing those in the health care ministry who often wear white, confirms this truth:

> It is only by knowing Jesus—not knowing about Jesus as an historical figure, but knowing Jesus through an encounter of prayer, where we welcome Jesus into our heart—that we find the motivation and power to imitate His selfless love.[149]

Spiritual formation, an encounter with the living God in Jesus and sustaining that personal relationship through prayer, the sacraments, Church teaching, and dialogue with fellow leaders are central ways to renew Catholic health care in all of its complexity in our world today. Delbecq and his co-authors see spiritual formation as central to the formation of Catholic institutional leaders: "Mission and Identity programs in

---

148 Daniel P. Sulmasy, "Without Love, We Perish," *Health Progress* (July–August 2009), 33.

149 Joseph F. Naumann, "The encounter with the Living God is the foundation of Christian medical practice," *The Linacre Quarterly* 83 (3) (2016), 237.

Catholic Healthcare are seen as a form of 'Spiritual Formation' separate from other arenas of leadership education and skill development."[150]

The desired outcome of these mission formation and identity programs is the transformation or the complete conversion (*metanoia*, or spiritual transformation in Christ) of the individual leader whose spiritual transformation will help him or her to become a spiritual leader for everyone in Catholic health care ministry from managers, to physicians, to staff, to patients, and those who encounter the healing mission of the Catholic facility. Delbecq and his co-authors state, "For Catholic institutions, we believe spiritual formation needs to be rooted in the Christian tradition that gave birth to and continues to sustain its ministries of healthcare, education and social services."[151]

The future of Catholic health care as a ministry in and of the Catholic Church depends upon leaders who can continue to steward and create cultures that know and love Jesus and inculcate his healing presence in their institutions and care, all the while providing expert and competent medical care. The ideal of Catholic health care ministry, as a ministry of the Church, O'Connell states, will be to form "organizational leaders who can articulate the identity and mission of Catholic

---

150 Delbecq, *Formation of Organizational Leaders*, 59.

151 Ibid., 59. Gerald Arbuckle has written a helpful book on the foundations of formation in Catholic health care titled, *Catholic Identity or Identities: Refounding Ministries in Chaotic Times*, which is a distilla-tion of what he considers core areas of competence and formation. He bases his concepts on the healing parables of Jesus and holistic healing. He also discusses the importance of Jesus as the founding principle of Catholic health care, not the mission of the Sisters. Gerald A. Arbuckle, *Catholic Identity or Identities: Refounding Ministries in Chaotic Times* (Collegeville, MN: Liturgical Press, 2013).

Health Care and integrate them into the complex, stratified work organization."[152]

Fr. Gerald Arbuckle has been prophetic in calling for renewed leadership formation in Catholic health care. He has called for it in many papers, lectures, and presentations, and has described it as something, I believe, akin to the needs of the new evangelization as called forth by Saint John Paul II.[153] The prophetic leader who is renewed and passionate about his or her relationship with Jesus must use new methods and visions for healing in the name of Christ. Arbuckle goes on to comment regarding the turbulence in Catholic health care: "Given such turmoil, Christ's healing mission will not be reenacted merely by polishing up—superficially improving or renewing—old methods of ministry and traditional methods of leadership. More radical responses will be necessary." Arbuckle foresees a new approach for health care leaders:

> Catholic health care will need the prophetic leadership qualities of its original founders. It will require people with similar imagination and creativity; people who, after first hearing and living the healing mission of Jesus Christ in their own lives, devise ways to reinterpret that mission for the turbulent, secularizing world of contemporary health care.[154]

---

152 O'Connell, *Tradition on the Move*, 30.

153 Pope John Paul II, as noted in chapter 2, spoke of how the new evangelization must include new methods, ardor, and vision in order to bring a renewed appreciation of the gift of faith. Catholic health care leaders must do the same so as to renew Jesus' mission of salvation and love in Catholic health care. See Pope John Paul II, Opening Address to the Assembly of CELAM, Port-au-Prince, Haiti, March 9, 1983.

154 Gerald A. Arbuckle, "Maintaining Prophetic Cultures," *Health*

During his visit to the United States in 2015, Pope Francis reminded Catholics to strive for a renewed focus on leadership of the Church's ministry:

> One of the great challenges facing the Church in this generation is to foster in all the faithful a sense of personal responsibility for the Church's mission, and to enable them to fulfill that responsibility as missionary disciples, as a leaven of the Gospel in our world.[155]

Thankfully, a number of Catholic health care systems have begun to develop leadership formation programs. In 2013, the first national study of all Catholic health care systems was conducted by the Center for Applied Research in the Apostolate, otherwise known as CARA. Many thought-provoking facts surfaced from this survey regarding formation of leaders and staff.

- Of the 64 systems that responded, most offered some type of formation program for leaders and ancillary staff. As Delbecq and co-authors comment: "With greater discretionary resources Catholic Healthcare, particularly the larger systems, have invested extensively in Mission and Identity formation in the last half decade."[156]

Progress (September–October 2005), 19-20.

155 Pope Francis, Homily at Mass, Cathedral of Sts. Peter and Paul, Philadelphia, Apostolic Journey to the United States, September 26, 2015. https://m.vatican.va/content/francesco/en/homilies/2015/documents/papa-francesco_20150926_usa-omelia-philadelphia.html (accessed on January 14, 2018).

156 Delbecq, *Formation of Organizational Leaders,* 58.

However, many smaller systems or stand-alone hospitals did not have the funds earmarked for formation programs for leadership.

- Most programs of formation were 12-23 months, and the second most popular length of formation was 24-35 months.

- The leadership formation programs offered a variety of formats.

- Most formation programs were offered within the system, although some formation occurred outside the system by using regional or national programs.

- Most formation programs were built around team and cohort models, while some included individual formation.

- In some cases, formation programs collaborated with other health care institutions and some educational or academic centers.[157]

Core Competencies for Catholic Health Care Leaders

Defining core competencies for the formation of leaders is essential. Most Sponsoring Systems have begun to define and articulate specific core competencies, which they believe are

---

157 Brian P. Smith and Sr. Patricia Talone, "Preliminary Results: CHA Survey Gauges Formation Effectiveness," *Health Progress*, (July-August 2014), 44-49.

necessary for the continued strengthening of Catholic health care. In identifying the core competencies (i.e., essential knowledge required of leaders), there were many similar themes. The Catholic Health Association, in its "Framework for Senior Leadership Formation," identified ten core areas of competence:

1. Heritage

2. Tradition and sponsorship

3. Mission and values

4. Vocation

5. Spirituality and theological reflection

6. Catholic social teaching

7. Ethics

8. Leadership style

9. Holistic health care

10. Diversity and church relations[158]

Delbecq and his co-authors, writing on the formation of Catholic leaders, identified 11 topics related to the field of

---

158 Ibid., 46. It is interesting to note that the authors speak of "ethics" rather than "moral theology." Moral theology helps in the right understanding of medical moral actions whereas ethics deals with how to choose what procedure might be most advantageous for the patient. The secular ethics may not always be grounded in Catholic moral theology. Also, there seems to be a lack of "theological anthropology" in the list. In other words why a particular treatment is proper to the human person who is created in the image and likeness of God and to return to God. Also, the theological foundations listed seem to be in short supply, except for the vague reference to "spirituality." In their listing, there is no explicit reference to Jesus Christ.

Catholic health care and Catholic education, which include many topics similarly identified in CHA's national survey from 2013.[159]

OSF HealthCare Ministry Leadership Formation Program

One system that has been on the forefront of formation of leaders and staff is the Sisters of the Third Order of St. Francis of East Peoria, Illinois, who operate OSF HealthCare based in Peoria, Illinois. OSF, as it will be referred to, has been a leader in ministry development for many years.

For more than 30 years, OSF has developed and earmarked funds for several effective formation programs for their employees. The Ministry Development Program began in 1989 in order to form leaders and key personnel throughout the system. The Sisters who realized they needed disciples of Jesus to continue the mission invited these individuals into formation. The Ministry Development program was created to form lay hospital leadership when the number of Sisters in leadership began to decline. The Ministry Development Program was a more general training program consisting of three main topics and lasted only one year with three retreats. These first leaders were trained by the sisters, as was explained in almost all the literature describing this transition from Religious leadership to lay leadership. The beginning formation was an immersion

---

159 Delbecq identifies these 11 topics as central to forming organizational leaders for Catholic mission and identity: Theological foundations, founders' stories as manifestation of the healing ministry of Jesus, vocation, spirituality, Catholic social teaching, organizational norms, dealing with diversity, ethics, ecclesiology and collaboration as participants in a ministry of the Church, mystery of suffering, and characteristic causes of distortions away from mission and values.

in the Catholic ethos, including the social teachings of the Church as well as the ERD's in the early 1980s.

As Catholic health care expanded to a growing population, and realizing that the Ministry Development Program could not have the desired effect of creating the intense and lasting formation that was needed for future health care leaders, the Sisters established a richer and more intense Christ-centered program, which they named the Ministry Leadership Formation Program (MLFP), MLFP was developed during the 1990s to form middle management, managers of departments, and people of principal influence, such as human resource directors. The program has expanded to more than 800 people employed in the Catholic health care ministry at OSF who are intentionally formed in the Catholic Church's health care mission. MLFP identifies a number of areas of core competence for formation, similar to the eleven CHA categories defined by Delbecq and his co-authors.

Sr. Judith Ann Duvall, chairperson of the OSF HealthCare System, said of the MLFP: "Being faithful to what God asks of us in OSF has so much more to do with who we are as persons than what we do or accomplish. In fact who we are is what drives the effectiveness of all we engage and nothing else."[160] As with all effective mission programs, it must be God who is the guiding force of what those, especially in Catholic health care, do. The Holy Spirit is the power from on high who fortifies and guides the actions of those who heal as they imitate Jesus, who became man to show us how to offer healing and love. OSF is particularly Trinitarian in its approach to

---

160 OSF, *Receiving His Grace through Formation*, Ministry Leadership Formation Publications, 2013, 3. OSF's MLFP is unpublished at this time.

forming leaders to recognize that God—as Father, Son, and Holy Spirit—is the center of all creation and wholeness. Their program of formation states in its introduction:

> We are leaders in Formation, an on-going journey in which we grow our faith and center our service within the foundation of Trinitarian Love. We are guided by the Holy Spirit to live more completely with God and serve others through Christ. Our service is an extension of God's love... We move beyond secular understanding of servant leadership to 'Service is Love.'[161]

Another feature of the MLFP at OSF is that it is "particularly brown," referring to the brown habits worn by those of the Third Order Regular of St. Francis. The heritage of OSF is Franciscan, and it examines its mission and work through the life and example of St. Francis of Assisi (1181-1226). The Franciscan spirit is what animated the Sisters' care from its beginning foundation in the late 1800's and still influences its ministry today, more than a hundred years later. The MLFP at OSF is based on a three-year sequence of formation of 5-7 formal teaching events each year, culminating in a capstone project[162] and Celebration Day in which participants are sent

---

161 Ibid., 3. Ascension Health, a mid-west Catholic health care system, began its leadership formation program in 2003 "in direct response to the Ascension Health vision for an increased role for the laity in the leadership and sponsorship of the Catholic healthcare ministry." This information is found in an unpublished article by Bill Brinkmann, Vice President for Mission Initiatives at Ascension Health. Request a copy at wbrinkmann@ascensionhealth.org.

162 Some examples of "capstone" projects have included such noteworthy topics as "Integrating a Mission and Values Guiding Principle into Prioritizing IT Projects;" "Developing a Call to Re-Connect Mini Retreat for Employees on Staff for 3-5 Years;" "Linking Community

forth into the OSF system to continue the Church's apostolate of healing.

Given that many leaders and others who are partners in Catholic health care are not Catholic or have no knowledge of the Catholic faith, sacraments, traditions, or heritage, it is essential that formation programs be especially clear in their expectations of Catholic identity and mission so that all people who are invited and charged with this tremendously important mission can share in promoting the love and healing of Jesus in Catholic health care.

Conclusion: Hope for the Future

As we have seen, the challenges to Catholic health care are numerous. There will always be a need to raise up and form prophetic voices who will embrace and champion the mission of Catholic health care. Our secular culture has little tolerance for Catholic Christian truths. An editorial in the *New York Times* stated:

> Freedom of religion is essential—and so is access to health care. Current law tries to accommodate both, but the far right has stirred unfounded fears that religion (and Christianity in particular) is under assault, and that people of faith are in danger of being forced to do things they find morally objectionable. "Patient-centered care" is an important goal in clinical training today, but the [presidential] administration is instead proposing provider-centered care.[163]

Health Needs Assessment to Care for the Homeless and Marginalized," to name just a few.

163 Editorial Board, "The White House Puts the Bible Before the

This mistaken belief that Catholic health care is opposed to "patient-centered care" is misguided and seems to imply that Catholic health care does not respect the autonomy of the person. What the *New York Times* and many others mistakenly assume is that whatever a person asks for in regard to his or her health, he or she should expect to receive, because it is his or her right as an individual. The Church's vision of health care does respect the autonomy of the patient, while keeping in mind the overall good and the rights of the professional staff and the health care institution. Our current culture can often be in direct conflict with the Catholic understanding of personal autonomy and may eventually prevent Catholic health care institutions from continuing their extraordinary legacy of care. External challenges to Catholic health care (e.g., the contraceptive mandate, government intrusion), internal challenges, and the decreased roles of leadership of consecrated religious have occasioned a new vision of lay leaders intentionally formed in Christ for strengthening Catholic health care in the United States.

The Church's vision for Catholic health care is guided by the love of Jesus Christ and each baptized disciple's call to proclaim the saving name of Jesus. Humans are meant to glorify God in their bodies. Moreover, each person's health is a gift from God, and thus it is an element of one's personal vocation to care for one's health. The Church will continue to offer health care because it is centered on the person who is made in the image and likeness of God and called to redemption.

The early religious were visionary, prophetic, and graced by

Hippocratic Oath," *The New York Times*, January 28, 2018. https://www. nytimes.com/2018/01/28/opinion/editorials/white-house-religious-freedom-doctors.html (accessed on January 29, 2018).

the Holy Spirit to see a need and meet it in the name of Christ. They were motivated by love to care for those who needed the love of God the most. The love which, they generously was demonstrated through the loving care of the Sisters and the best-known medical practice of the time. They served all those who came to them, regardless of their illness, religion, color, or status. They served in imitation of Jesus's saving love for all. They built Catholic hospitals, schools, orphanages, and other institutions for the purpose of caring for others as a ministry in and with the Church. The early religious in this country came at the requests of bishops and priests to serve immigrant populations, victims of disease, the poor, and outcast. As they continued to serve with the greatest love, their Catholic hospitals and health care institutions expanded to meet the need of a growing population in the United States.

During the early 1970s, as the number of consecrated religious in hospital leadership began to decline, the role of ministry was handed on to lay men and women, who because of their baptism in Christ, shared in the role of ministry within the Church. Lay leadership began to expand at a rapid pace with very little formal training or formation. This occasioned a weakening of the Catholic identity and mission in Catholic health care. Mergers and buyouts also caused confusion, and religious sponsors, who once defined the leadership roles for the purpose of handing on this sacred mission, became separated from this role and influence in forming leaders in their charism and the ministry of Catholic health care. With the absence of strong formation programs, Catholic identity was no longer a priority for many leaders and the connection to the local Church, through the bishop, became distant.

There is reason for hope, however, for the future ministry

of Catholic health care, because enhanced formation programs for leaders will strengthen and bolster this heritage of Catholic health care. Well-defined and enhanced formation programs will assist Catholic health care leaders in embracing the life and outreach of Jesus in their ministry in Catholic health care. The Pontifical Council remarks:

> The new evangelization, therefore, does not necessarily require the invention of something new to be done, but, rather, the promotion and strengthening in all believers of a common and shared vision of reality which springs from faith, and which in its turn generates a "new" way of thinking about human life and a new way of acting toward it in relation to everything that concerns it and which is very different to what the dominant secularized culture says about it.[164]

The emphasis on living the new evangelization will embolden leaders to embrace a new way of ministering, caring for, and serving God's people. This new ardor that leaders display will come about through an increased and deepened relationship with Jesus. As leaders experience the healing power and love of Jesus, they too, with ongoing formation, will grow in that love of service of others and bring about change in their policies, formation of other staff, and become an example to the people they serve. Through an embrace of their baptismal dignity, Catholic health care leaders will

---

164 The Pontifical Council for Health Care Workers, *Pastoral Care in Health and the New Evangelization for the Transmission of the Faith*, 41-42. Both Pope Saint John Paul II and Pope Francis point to the dignity and enhanced respect for the human person that Catholic health care brings to the topic of a renewed Catholic health care.

respond to the original call of healing with Christ-like love, which the early religious carried out in the name of the Church.

What the new evangelization can offer to Catholic health care is a renewed energy, purpose, and deepening of the Gospel message of love and compassion. Jesus fully lived this message in his day-to-day care of the poor, the outcast, and the sick and infirm, and those who believed they were unlovable.

The focus of those in leadership in Catholic health care is to show Jesus' love to a world so desperately in need of it. The Fathers of the Second Vatican Council wanted to convey to the world, especially in *Gaudium et Spes* and *Lumen Gentium*, that the Church has something so valuable and so life-giving to say to a world that wants to eliminate its voice. O'Connell writes to this concern: "Its mission (the Church's) is to be a seed of transformation in the larger culture. It calls the culture to persist in the paths that maximize human well-being and models a way of serving that is meant to show the true potential of every human being and community."[165] Catholic health care is not about retreating from the world; it is about engaging the world with Jesus' healing love. Daniel Sulmasy speaks to the importance of the Church's spiritual grounding in health care in an interview he gave to a Catholic publication:

> This talk has more to do with a call for us to return to a fundamentally Christian orientation toward the world, with seeing Jesus' washing of the feet of the disciples as normative, with understanding that if we name a hospital after the Good Samaritan that we ought to start behaving as if we believed that these stories

---

165 O'Connell, *Tradition on the Move*, 49.

about the meaning of love were the true meaning of all ethics.[166]

What Sulmasy is identifying is the call to return to Catholic health care as a ministry of Jesus. Jesus' ministry was a ministry of healing and serving the poor, the suffering, and the sick in order to lead to the recognition that the saving Kingdom of God was in their midst. The ERDs state it most directly:

> The mystery of Christ casts light on every facet of Catholic health care: to see Christian love as the animating principle of health care; to see healing and compassion as a continuation of Christ's mission; to see suffering as a participation in the redemptive power of Christ's passion, death, and resurrection; and to see death, transformed by the resurrection, as an opportunity for a final act of communion with Christ.[167]

Catholic health care has continued this type of care and desires to carry it out more robustly in the future. The Church, including Catholic hospitals, parishes, and institutions that live this message, will show the negative voices in the world that Catholic health care truly desires the integral good of the patient. Pope Francis has reiterated this same call for the whole Church to embrace each individual, especially the marginalized and the outcast. He remarked in his message for the World Day of the Sick in 2018:

> The Church's mission is a response to Jesus' gift, for she

---

166 Sulmasy, "Without Love, We Perish," 34.

167 *Ethical and Religious Directives*, General Introduction, 3.

knows that she must bring to the sick the Lord's own gaze, full of tenderness and compassion. Health care ministry will always be a necessary and fundamental task, to be carried out with renewed enthusiasm by all, from parish communities to the largest healthcare institutions.[168]

What Pope Francis is echoing is the Church's long held concern for the spiritual and physical healing of all people. The Church has fulfilled this mission in Catholic health care first envisioned by dedicated religious who invited the laity into this same ministry as fellow baptized followers in Christ. The Holy Father confirms that the mission of Catholic health care belongs to all in the Church as a "shared responsibility that enriches the value of daily service given by each [member]."[169]

Formation of all who minister in Catholic health care, especially leadership development, is critical to the continued mission of the Church. If those in Catholic health care are going to minister to others, both physically and (most importantly) spiritually, then they have to help the world to see the person-centered love that Jesus has for the defenseless young to the elderly. Our care must be grounded in a deep love and concern for the inalienable dignity of each human person. Sulmasy brings home this point:

Christian health care must be based on love, and love is not an abstraction. Love is concrete. We will need

168 Pope Francis, "Message of His Holiness Pope Francis for the Twenty-Sixth World Day of the Sick 2018." https://w2.vatican.va/content/francesco/en/messages/sick/documents/papa-francesco_20171126_giornata-malato.html (accessed on January 30, 2018).

169 Pope Francis, "World Day of the Sick 2018."

programs. We will need skilled administration. We will need extraordinary physicians and nurses and chaplains and social workers and patient transporters and lab technicians. But unless all of this is pursued in love, it will come to nothing.[170]

Formation not only for leaders, but also for all who participate in the mission of Catholic health care, must provide a personal encounter with Jesus, the divine physician, in ongoing and sustained formation. Our goal is that all who come to Catholic health care institutions to be healed will experience Christ's saving love.

There is cause for hope in this future as many religious sponsors of hospital systems and health care organizations are responding to the need for leadership formation and ministry development in Catholic health care. As Pope Francis, Daniel Sulmasy, and others argue, Catholic health care is distinct and of value, precisely because it is based on divine love. God's love in Jesus must be the animating principle of all we do in Catholic health care. Healing love, perfectly modeled only by Christ, is what inspired the Sisters and it is what must inspire all mission partners in Catholic health care today.

Thankfully, many hospitals and sponsoring organizations are taking concrete steps in the formation of lay leaders. The original religious sisters who led the hospitals are no longer actively engaged in leadership, and those they trained are nearing retirement. The current leaders or soon-to-be leaders

---

170 Sulmasy, "*Without Love, We Perish,*" 35. 1 Corinthians 13 is the goal and reason for the Church's ministry in health care. Sulmasy goes on to comment that the religion, which established our hospitals, was founded on an encounter with the God who is love (1 John 4:8). "That encounter must be the foundation of our health care systems and our institutions." Sulmasy, *Without Love, We Perish,*" 33.

have been more influenced by our secular and pluralistic society than the Catholic ethos that surrounded our Catholic hospitals previously. Archbishop Zygmunt Zimowski, President of the Pontifical Council for Pastoral Care Workers, named this threat when he said that:

> ... this new Charter for Health Care Workers, [which] is meant to be an effective tool for confronting the weakening of ethical standards and the subjectivity of consciences which, together with cultural, ethical, and religious pluralism, easily lead to relativism and hence to the risk that we will no longer be able to refer to a shared ethos, especially in regard to the major existential questions pertaining to the meaning of birth, life, and death.[171]

It is first and foremost the responsibility of the sponsoring congregations to make formation a significant and vital element for new leaders. Sponsoring organizations, with the help of Catholic educational facilities or other institutions with proven records of rich theological and extensive formation, should partner with Catholic health care institutions in forming the next generation of leaders to further the mission of the Church. The formation of leaders must include at least a two- or three-year program of formation to ensure proficiency in core competencies, as well as ongoing formation, which should include a capstone project to tie all the formation together. Formation must also include time for leaders to experience

---

171 Pontifical Council for Pastoral Assistance to Health Care Workers, *New Charter for Health Care Workers*, The National Catholic Bioethics Center: Philadelphia, PA, 2016, viii.

Jesus as savior and Lord and to see how his love can be put into practice in their ministry and leadership.

Catholic health care leaders and sponsors must also be willing to deepen and fortify their relationship with the Church, as a minister of her apostolate, through the diocesan bishop. This should include at least quarterly contact with the diocesan bishop, creating a shared vision, and receiving feedback on the direction and goals being accomplished in Catholic health care in the name of the Church. Creating or renewing this relationship will allow the Catholic health care facility to build that necessary relationship with the bishop, parishes, and other churches and ecclesial communions so as to enhance the means of evangelization for the community, as well as those whose ministry is Catholic health care. I believe this renewed relationship with the Church, as represented by the bishop, is a key component for the future ministry of Catholic health care.

Zeni Fox, in writing of the future of lay leaders and the mission of Catholic health care, makes the point that the Church, in her ministries properly guided and formed, can continue to make a difference for good in the world. She argues:

> The constant touchstone for the lay leader must be the mission of the institution, with its priority given to human flourishing. An internal organization culture that keeps its priorities straight and combines a strong faith commitment with delivery of excellent services to its constituencies holds something essential for the culture beyond itself: it proclaims, in its daily activities, that it is possible to be religious and a servant of the

wider culture and its needs, to be faith-oriented and competent.[172]

As was referred to in the previous chapters, Catholic health care is undergoing rapid change, both inside its halls as well as outside. Pope Francis stated that we will always need Catholic health care, and renewed formation is a key to its revitalization and future success. Lawrence O'Connell, in his work in leadership formation, summarizes the issue:

> The community of Catholic Health Care is undergoing two waves of change. One wave is internal: the numerical decline and repositioning of the religious women who carried the responsibility for Catholic identity and mission. The other wave is the change in U.S. health care, of which Catholic Health Care is a part. This change has many facets, all of which have some impact on the range and content of formation. But the overall impact is the emergence of organizational bigness and business complexity. Both these waves represent dangers and opportunities. Catholic identity and mission may be lost or they may find new and more effective contemporary forms. It is this open future that pushes Catholic Health Care into the arduous task of becoming a formation organization.[173]

Zeni Fox's comment is a clear expression of the exciting challenges God is asking us to take on and the careful planning

---

172 Fox, *Called & Chosen*, 96.

173 O'Connell, *Tradition on the Move*, 29.

for the future we must engage in if we are going to fulfill the Church's vision of Catholic health care in a new world.

New questions regarding partnership, cooperation, and for-profit and not-for-profit status in Catholic health care will need to be continually addressed and reviewed by leaders, sponsors, diocesan bishops, and others charged with its mission.[174] There may come a time when competent authorities require that particular Catholic health care institutions, which are not abiding by Catholic teaching because of a merger or buy out, have their Catholic identity revoked.[175] The ERDs can and will continue to be a necessary tool in guiding and forming all people involved in Catholic health care.

What will continue to distinguish Catholic health care from other medical care is the love of Jesus, which guides and inspires all those involved in its ministry. From the formation of its leaders and partners in the rich understanding of God's love in Jesus Christ, loving care will continue to make an impact on those who are served in Catholic health care and those who minister in Jesus' name. Therese Lysaught's insightful book states the following in regard to Catholic identity:

> Catholic health care is a concrete practice of love. It takes shape as a communion of people engaged in ministry and witness, steeped in Catholic social thought and the Spirit-led charisms of our founders,

---

174 See the revised sixth edition of the *Ethical and Religious Directives for Catholic Health Care Services*, Part VI promulgated by the United States Bishops in June 2018.

175 See the *Seattle Times* article on Bishop Robert Vasa's decision to remove St. Charles Hospitals' Catholic status because of their persistence in performing tubal ligations. https://www.seattletimes.com/seattle-news/oregon-diocese-severs-ties-with-hospital/ (accessed on January 19, 2018).

which continue to inspire our ministry. Catholic health care is sacramental, grounded in an ecclesiology rooted in Christ, the summit and fullness of God's caritas in the world.[176]

Lysaught conveys what can happen when Catholic health care leaders understand that their formation in care and compassion is ultimately directed toward the gift of salvation Jesus came to offer every person.

The Church has a profound opportunity to evangelize in the field of Catholic health care through its training and formation of leaders. These leaders have the opportunity to transform a whole culture of people, patients, medical staff, and the community by the way they carry out their ministry in the name of the Church. Many sponsors and organizations host professional development days for health care leaders; they also need to provide retreat days and intense periods of formation directed toward proclaiming the new evangelization. Pope Saint Paul VI in his profound and often quoted apostolic exhortation states, "The task of evangelizing all people constitutes the essential mission of the Church."[177]

Catholic health care is in a privileged position to evangelize, to bring Christ's healing love to the world through its Spirit-led, medically excellent, and charitable caring. Lay leaders and all the laity in Catholic health care have a privileged

---

176 Lysaught, *Caritas in Communion: Theological Foundations of Catholic Health Care* (St. Louis, MO: Catholic Health Association, 2014), 121. Her study covers a vast array of Catholic health care studies and practices, which she has participated in and witnessed first-hand. Her book speaks deeply to the need for those in Catholic health care to have a strong sense of community in Christ, and thus a community of love.

177 Pope Paul VI, *Evangelii Nuntiandi*, 14.

opportunity to renew the hospital culture for Christ. Ministry leadership formation programs must be developed promptly to form lay leaders in their essential role of bringing about the new evangelization in Catholic health care. This can happen only by their embrace of and witness to Jesus Christ.

Personal Faith Formation of Leaders

If the Catholic health care mission and the life of holiness to which Jesus calls all the baptized is developed and deepened within health care leaders, their outlook and way of addressing issues in their institution will lead to spiritual growth within themselves and within the organization. A Christ-like perspective that will begin to change the health care culture from the top down will mark how the leaders respond to challenges—including the spiritual, personal, and financial—. Once formation programs are implemented with individual leaders, such as managers, vice-presidents, mission coordinators, human resource leaders, and board members, the *metanoia* of the individual leader can lead in the transformation of the hospital culture. When these commonly held Christ-centered beliefs are lived out by the health care leaders, it will lead to the increased promotion of the mission and the strengthening of the facilities' fidelity to the mission of Jesus, the Church and its Catholic founders.

Formation of lay leaders in the person, life, and teaching of Jesus, as a response to their baptismal call, cannot be accomplished by one formation program presented by a sponsoring religious sister. Formation must include competencies in the comprehensive teachings of the Church related to Catholic health care and its mission in the world.

Competencies that are essential are Catholic social teaching, Catholic health care ethics, moral theology, Sacred

Scripture, the documents of the Second Vatican Council, Vatican and Congregational documents on the topic of Catholic health care, and documents issued by the USCCB, particularly the ERDs. Formation must be consistent, ongoing, and deepen each year so that lay health care leaders, sharing in the apostolate of the Church, will be sustained for ministry to all people of the world. As O'Connell wrote in regard to formation:

> [Catholic health care leaders] have the credentials and skills to do the work in their area of expertise and this makes them marketable in the health [care] world. But, at this moment, their organization has invited them into a formation experience that is designed to bring them into greater alignment with the Catholic identity and mission. The sequence of this formation path is through work understood as part of personal life into formation—at a certain point in their careers and at the request of the organization that presently employs them—to become more deeply aligned with the organizational mission, vision, and values that are informed and sponsored by a faith-based community/ tradition.[178]

Just as the formation of priests, religious, and deacons has a defined course of study approved by the Church, so too should the stewards of the Church's healing ministry be formed in a defined manner according to the mind and heart of the Church. Catholic health care leaders will be better assisted by entering into a formation program designed to help them to encounter Jesus and his call to go forth and minister to the

178 O'Connell, *Tradition on the Move*, 65.

sick and downtrodden. O'Connell sees formation as akin to how the religious were trained: "some voices suggest that the formation path of women religious is normative" in Catholic health care.[179]

CHA and many others have commented on the necessity of leadership formation: "Each system must determine how to offer formation according to its economic reality; however, not to offer any leadership formation, or just [to offer] a module now and then, is not being a good steward of the value of the Catholic health care ministry."[180] We have been speaking of the apostolate of Jesus and his Church in the world. Given today's rampant secularism, to not offer any formation could be considered a grave moral evil since one does not make Jesus' mission the focus. In fact, a study conducted by Arbuckle found that out of 25 Catholic health care institutions, only 12 mentioned the name of Jesus in their mission statement.[181] As was commented on earlier, this lack of Christ-centered focus is a real concern.

The failure of a Catholic health care organization to offer formation would also seem to be a sin against charity because one does not give one's neighbor what he or she needs most: Christ's saving love. Not only is ministry leadership formation a necessity, it could also be an example for other Catholic institutions facing leadership challenges in the future.[182]

179 Ibid., 63.

180 Smith, *CHA Survey Gauges Formation Effectiveness*, 5.

181 Arbuckle, *Catholic Identity or Identities*, 83.

182 See Delbecq and his co-authors' excellent article on the "Formation of Organizational Leaders for Catholic Mission and Identity," especially in the section titled, "Relevance of the Healthcare Formation Experience to Higher Education," pp. 69-71.

An article summarizing CHA's survey on formation effectiveness showed that there is multiple ways formation is being delivered. Not all systems have the resources to develop their own programs, so some are collaborating with other Catholic health systems and universities. Because leadership formation is considered important for other Catholic ministries, such as higher education, Catholic social service agencies, and diocesan ministries, is there possible collaboration for lay ministry formation programs that might serve a variety of Catholic ministries? This could be especially useful for small Catholic systems and stand-alone or rural facilities. Other Catholic ministries already look to Catholic health care's model of formation as a possible framework they can adopt.[183]

Ongoing formation must be an area where resources are invested if Catholic health care is going to continue to be a mission of Jesus and his Church. In speaking of the necessity of continued formation in Catholic health care for the future, O'Connell states the charge this way: "In fact, the people and the services are so intimately linked, so interdependent with one another, that it is impossible to conceive of the services without conceiving of people who are formed in a certain way to provide them."[184] Michael Downey, writing about lay and institutional spirituality in the formation of leaders, states:

> In sum: The lay leader must have (1) competence in the enterprise at hand; (2) a deep passion for the enterprise and the persons served by it, as well as for those who, together with the leader, serve it; and (3) a facility for communication of a specific Christian vision to

183 Smith, *CHA Survey Gauges Formation Effectiveness*, 45.

184 O'Connell, *Tradition on the Move*, 53.

one's colleagues and collaborators, as well as to the constituents of the other worlds of meaning, purpose, and value of which one's enterprise is a part. This is the Spirit's gift, enlightening, enlivening, and guiding the leader to ponder long and lovingly, giving shape to a vision of the reign of God at this time and in this place, thereby participating in the mission of Word and Spirit for the transformation of the whole world and all the living in and through love.[185]

I believe Downey's summary of what a leader's vision should be in Catholic health care is clearly articulated in his three statements. Although there are varying interpretations of what should be considered a core competency, especially for the formation of Catholic health care leaders, I believe that the core competencies mentioned here within this book provide more than sufficient grounding in the mission of healing first given by Jesus and carried out in Catholic health care in the past and to today. As Arbuckle comments, "It is not the tradition of the Sisters that is to be the primary concern in Catholic healthcare, but the healing mission of Jesus Christ."[186]

Ministry Formation:
A Personal Encounter With Jesus

Being actively involved in Catholic health care in the nine Catholic hospitals and one ecumenical facility, which adheres

---

185 Michael Downey, "'Without a Vision the People Perish': Foundations for a Spirituality of Lay Leadership," in *Called & Chosen*, ed. Zeni Fox and Regina Bechtle (Lanham, MD: Rowman & Littlefield Publishers, 2005), 28.

186 Gerald A. Arbuckle, *Catholic Identity or Identities: Refounding Ministries in Chaotic Times* (Minneapolis, MN: Liturgical Press, 2013), 83.

to the ERD's, in the Diocese of Peoria has afforded me rich opportunities for evaluating programs geared toward the evangelization of health care leaders. I have participated in numerous weekend retreats as well as conferences that have focused on the formation of health care leaders. The *Audits* of our nine Catholic hospitals and one ecumenical facility have allowed me to see firsthand the ease with which our mission can be lost without ongoing intentional formation programs.[187] It has also made me keenly aware of the necessity of good leadership formation for the renewal of Catholic health care according to the principles of the new evangelization as envisioned by the Church.

After studying and working in the field of Catholic health care since 2000, I have found that the most successful formation programs contain four main elements:

1. The period of formation must be ongoing. I discovered, along with other findings, that a three-year period has been the most effective in creating a real encounter between Jesus and the participant. A continued three-year emphasis allows the relationship cultivated in Christ at the beginning of formation to be deepened and therefore sustained over the next number of years.

2. Formation in core competencies is essential to fully

---

187 The Diocese of Peoria, 28 years ago, instituted audits, patterned after the Joint Commission, process whereby Catholic facilities are reviewed for upholding Catholic moral teaching and the guidelines of the ERD's. It was also an opportunity to build a relationship with hospital leadership and the diocesan bishop through his delegate. See my article on "Catholic Health Care Audits" in *Ethics & Medics* (April 2011), Vol. 36, No. 4.

grasp the nature and purpose of Catholic health care as envisioned by Jesus. The core competencies I propose include the tradition of Catholic health care, the healing miracles of Jesus described in the scriptures, the legacy and charism of the founders, the mission of the Church and the role of the laity, Catholic health care as an apostolate of the Church and the role of the local bishop, the social doctrine of the Church, and care for the poor and outcast.

3. Regular spiritual encounters with the Lord must be included in formation so that each participant can have an encounter with the Lord's healing and presence in their own lives. Such encounters include personal prayer, reception of the Sacraments, Eucharist Adoration, directed retreats, silence and meditation, and daily moments of reflection and sharing.

4. After the three-year period of intense formation, ongoing formation, education, and retreats designed to keep the mission-oriented focus before the health care leader must continue. There must be a frequent emphasis on teaching the message and on the lived experience of each of the leaders, lest they become a "noisy gong or a clanging symbol" (1 Cor. 13:1), as St. Paul says of those who do not live out the value of Christ-like love.

Conclusion

It is exciting to see an increased focus and interest in the formation of Catholic health care leaders. If we were to review a representative sample of sponsoring organizations—such as Catholic Health Initiatives, OSF HealthCare, Ascension Health, Catholic Health East, and the Ministry Leadership Center—one would notice that many sizeable systems are recognizing the need to establish formation programs for health care leaders. It is from this sampling of programs that I am hopeful for the continued flourishing of Catholic health care in accord with its mission. It is also exciting to see many formation programs established in Catholic health care partnering with Catholic educational facilities—the National Catholic Bioethics Center, Loyola University of Chicago, St. Louis University in St. Louis, Missouri, and Georgetown to name just a few— to provide common modules of training that could assist the Church and the bishops in this most necessary mission. It is interesting to note that all of the Catholic medical schools in the United States are Jesuit institutions and is linked to Jesuit educational facilities. If Catholic educational institutions already have established methods for forming educational leaders, it would make sense to incorporate ministry formation programs for health care leadership within this Catholic framework of formation. As more and more systems merge, it would be also be advantageous to develop a systematic program of formation coordinated by the U.S. bishops in collaboration with an already established and trusted formation program, such as the National Catholic Bioethics Center (NCBC). The NCBC offers an excellent certification program that could be the beginning format for all Catholic health care staff. I hope to see the day when this idea of a coordinated formation program in core competencies in Catholic health care becomes a reality for the Church in the United States and its mission of Catholic health care.

Ministry formation must be an essential part of the future of Catholic health care, especially if Catholic health care is going to continue as an authentic mission of the Church. If hospital systems and those responsible for them do not make this a priority, Catholic health care may find itself in an identity crisis with the result being increased secularization in both its ministers and ministry. Mission formation programs must be developed and sustained to form leaders in the core competencies. These core competencies will then ground Catholic health care leaders in understanding the Church's legacy of Catholic health care so they can evangelize the world for Christ through their ministry. As Lawrence O'Connell predicts, "Ministry formation for twenty-first century leaders requires reflection and experimentation on many fronts. The restless tradition of Catholic Health Care inspires us to find better ways to care for one another."[188]

A Module of Leadership Formation

Ministry leadership formation is essential to the future of Catholic health care. Catholic health care sponsors, faced with the decline in their numbers as Consecrated Religious, have had to pass on the torch to lay leaders in an era when the laity have been called upon to assume greater responsibility for the transmission of the Faith. Delbecq remarks:

The development of a spiritual formation program

---

188 O'Connell, *Tradition on the Move*, xi.

within an organization creates a path on which participants can deepen their awareness of how they are being formed, can be intentional about choosing formational practices, and can welcome the active presence of the Divine, who accomplishes more in and among the group than planners and facilitators can envision.[189]

To continue the ministry of Catholic health care, it is necessary to ground formation in a number of core principles as was mentioned in Chapter Four. I propose seven core principles to ensure that the next generation of Catholic health care leaders will be able to continue and sustain a thriving apostolate for the Church:

1. The healing miracles of Jesus as described in the sacred Scriptures

2. The tradition of Catholic health care

3. The legacy and charism of the original founders of the health care institution

4. The mission of the Church and the essential role of the laity in this mission

5. Catholic Health Care as an apostolate of the Church and the essential role of the Diocesan Bishop

6. The Social Doctrine of the Church

---

189 Delbecq, *Formation of Organizational Leaders for Catholic Mission and Identity*, 59.

7. The role of Catholic Health Care in serving the poor, the sick and the outcast

These seven competencies are essential and manageable components in a three-year formation program in developing leaders in Catholic health care and can provide the reasons for the belief and the mission. These seven core principles, I believe, provide a firm grounding and a reason for why Catholic health care existed in the past and why it must exist today in a renewed way. With a three-year program in mind, I propose that all seven of these topics can be covered in a three-year period. These competencies are all closely linked and connected so that in the three years of formation, each topic adds more specific layers and a deeper grounding of the Catholic health care leader in the complete ethos of healing as the Church understood the mandate from Jesus.

In this three-year formation process each year becomes the foundation for the next topics to establish grounding and meaning. Formation one weekend a month is the most suitable way for busy health care leaders to commit to this process of formation and to have the opportunity for deep and lasting growth in the spiritual riches of Catholic health care. The program of formation could begin Friday afternoon and conclude on Sunday afternoon, ideally once a month or if this becomes too difficult to manage, could be arranged to end Saturday evening. Each System coordinating this program of formation would have to determine what times and days are most feasible for the leader(s). Each weekend would involve reading pertinent information in preparation for the monthly weekend program. Following each conference throughout the weekend, participants would be expected to maintain a written journal and provide a one page review of how this topic applies to the Church's understanding of

Catholic health care and fits into their particular experience and outreach in Catholic health care at their facility.

The seven core principles are the topic headings of each of the three years of formation. The talks listed in italics would be the key topics to highlight in presenting talks directed at each of the key areas. These topics over a three-year cycle are outlined in the in the following paragraphs. Within this book, I have included another helpful resource for formation of Catholic Health Care leaders which is, *Appendix B: A Retreat Model for Health Care Leaders,* which defines even more clearly, the topics and talks that could be given.

Year One

Grounding in the healing ministry of Jesus' saving love as shown in his miracles and how the early religious accomplished this healing through their ministry and the particular charism, which inspired Christ-like healing.

Topics:

1. Old Testament and New Testament examples of healing

2. How the healings of Jesus made known/visible the Kingdom of God

3. Jesus is the incarnational love of the Fathers' love for all people.

4. By Jesus' incarnation, the entire world and those in it can be sanctified, restored and saved.

5. The early religious, inspired by Jesus and his saving

love, wanted to make this love present in their care for the poor, diseased, homeless, abandoned and ill

6. Catholic health care developed from the ministry of the early religious

7. Explanation and study of the particular charism of the Order/Founding Congregation

8. How this Catholic health care ministry operates today either alone or merged

9. Christ-like healing is at the core of Catholic health care

In the first year of formation, the curriculum includes a thorough scriptural study of Jesus' healing ministry and how Jesus' healings revealed and made visible the Kingdom of God. The formation continues developing the leaders' concept of how Jesus is at the center of this formation and the center of this love they are called to offer. This first year also includes a clear understanding of the concept that *Jesus is Lord and Savior and it is in His Incarnational Love that Catholic health care can make that love visible by the way they treat the sick.* Catholic health care is first and foremost about making Jesus' healing love known through competent care and Christ like presence through all involved. The first-year curriculum grounds leaders in *The Healing Miracles of Jesus and the Reason for His Coming; Awareness of the Past: A Recognition of the Founding Congregation and its Charisms*, and thirdly *The Spirituality of Healing at the Core.*

Suggested Readings:

Tobit 12

Matthew 8:1-4 "Healing of the Leper" and Mark 1:40-42

Matthew 20:29-34 "Man born blind."

John 6:35 and John 11:25-27

Luke 10:25-37 "The Good Samaritan"

Ministry & Meaning: A Religious History of Catholic Health Care in the United States by Christopher J. Kauffman. (See Bibliography)

Called to Serve: A History of Nuns in America by Margaret M. McGuinness (see Bibliography)

Jesus of Nazareth by Cardinal Josef Ratzinger

The Ethical and Religious Directives for Catholic Health Care Services: Preamble and Introduction

Article 5: The Anointing of the Sick [CCC 1499-1532]

Year Two

The Ministry of Catholic Health care as a work of the Church and the involvement of religious, laity, clergy and Bishops as envisioned by the Second Vatican Council for ministry to the world.

Topics:

1. How was the Catholic Church established? Why was it established?

2. How were the religious orders fulfilling the mission of Jesus through the Church in Catholic health care?

3. What was the role of the Bishop of the Diocese and the religious sisters?

4. The Second Vatican Council and its documents on the laity

5. How did the Church envision the laity being involved in evangelizing?

6. How were the laity involved and invited into Catholic health care?

7. What is the mission/apostolate of Catholic health care today, especially in light of the ERD's?

8. Is the Catholic health care institution advancing the Gospel message of Jesus?

9. Is the Catholic health care facility regularly engaged with the Bishop of the local diocese?

10. Is Catholic health care bringing Christ and the Lord's saving love to the people they minister too regardless of race, religion or color?

Suggested Readings:

Gaudium et Spes, 24, 31, 33, 40, 43

Lumen Gentium, 12, 30, 31

Apostolicam Acousitatem, 2, 4-8, 16, 28-32

The Ethical and Religious Directives for Catholic Health Care Services: Part One & Two

"The Charter for Health Care Workers" from the Vatican

"Formation of Organizational Leaders for Catholic Mission and Identity" by Andre L. Delbecq, Jack Mudd and Celeste Mueller (see Bibliography)

Vatican Expert Unpacks Canonical PJP Process by Sr. Sharon Holland, IHM

The Vocation to Heal: Health Care in the Light of Catholic Faith: Scriptural, Theological and Philosophical Reflections." By Mark Latkovic (see Bibliography)

Tradition on the Move: Leadership Formation in Catholic Health Care by Lawrence O'Connell and John Shea (see Bibliography)

In the second year of formation, the curriculum begins with the *Theological Grounding of Catholic Health Care.* It includes in-depth coverage of *The Ethical and Religious Directives for Catholic Health Care Services,* an excellent guide to follow in forming Catholic health care leaders. Next is *Connected to the Church: Catholic Health Care as an Apostolate of the Church,* which

118

links the ERDs to the healing power of Jesus and the Church's health care mission in close connection to the bishop and local diocese. This year also explores in depth the writings of the Fathers of the Second Vatican Council and its teachings in particular on the role of the laity in sanctifying the world, which applies particularly well to the field of Catholic health care.

Year Three

The implementation of Christ's healing love to the world through the Social Doctrine of the Church and those in need as an embodiment of Christian healing through leadership formation of all involved.

Topics:

1. What is the social doctrine of the Church?

2. Who carries it out today in the Church?

3. What is the role of the Church in caring for the poor and needy?

4. What is the Bishop's connection to Catholic health care today?

5. How can the Catholic health care facility cooperate with Catholic parishes and other Christian Communities?

6. How can Community Clinics bring Christ's healing love to the area?

7. What is the spiritual meaning of suffering as Jesus envisioned?

8. What about the responsibility of providing charity care?

9. Could the Catholic health facility partner with other facilities, Catholic or non-Catholic, to provide better and more complete care for all of Christ's faithful?

Suggested Readings:

Evangelii Gaudium by Pope Francis

Salvifici Dolores by Pope John Paul II

The Code of Canon Law, paragraphs 381 & 394

"A Big Heart Open to God: An Interview with Pope Francis" in America (see Bibliography)

Discerning the Future of the American Catholic Health Ministry by John A. Gallagher (see Bibliography)

Pontifical Council for Justice and Peace, "Compendium of the Social Doctrine of the Church," 2004.

Health and Health Care Pastoral Letter of US Bishops

The Ethical and Religious Directives for Catholic Health Care, Part IV

Sulmasy, Daniel P. "Without Love, We Perish: Gospel-Centered Health Care Is a Radical Approach in Today's Secular World." *Health Progress* (July–August 2009), 30-36

The third year of formation includes the mission of Catholic health care, namely *Catholic Health Care as Mission Oriented: Roles of Service.* The last topic is *Collaboration in the Church:*

Working With Other Health Care Organizations to build up Catholic health care while partnering with parishes, Catholic facilities, and Catholic educational institutions. The third year can also include a careful moral analysis of partnership opportunities with other Catholic facilities and institutions to bring about the best health care for the common good. An example of this is the cooperation with another facility to provide combined psychological or neurological services where shortages are creating crises for Catholic health care ministry.

Each topic is framed within a teachable session with plenty of opportunity for discussion and input. The program combines pedagogy with discipleship so that the topics are interwoven with practice. The three-year program also provides retreat moments to allow the Holy Spirit to speak to the hearts of those going through leadership formation. Jesus often went away by himself to pray, to commune with God the Father so that he could be filled more deeply with the presence and strength of God. Health care leaders will benefit by following this same model of discernment.

Delbecq again remarks:

> The development of a spiritual formation program within an organization creates a path on which participants can deepen their awareness of how they are being formed, can be intentional about choosing formational practices, and can welcome the active presence of the Divine, who accomplishes more in and among the group than planners and facilitators can envision.[190]

---

190 175 Delbecq, 59.

A Retreat Model for Catholic Health Care Leaders

As a way of assisting in the formation of Catholic health care leaders, I will share a weekend retreat module for health care leaders in the appendix. I hope the model presented will become a resource to help strengthen Catholic identity (and mission) in Catholic health care. The weekend retreat model is listed below.

This two-day formation retreat is for Catholic health care leaders who have 3-5 years of leadership experience in Catholic health care. The purpose of this retreat is to provide an opportunity for the health care leader to see his or her sacred role in the context of faith and to deepen his or her relationship with the Lord. Deepening this relationship with the Lord will fortify the Catholic health care leader to see his or her ministry as essentially connected with and directed toward the healing of people in the name of Christ Jesus.

A two-day retreat provides the opportunity for busy health care leaders to slow down, to allow God to speak to their hearts, and to provide the space to listen to his teaching. It is only when they quiet their hearts and minds and then learn to listen to the presentations, the Gospel reflections, the Holy Spirit, and Jesus that leaders can grow spiritually and then evangelize the world through Catholic health care.

The retreat includes three scripturally-based reflections on the healing parables of Jesus, catechetical teaching, explanation of Church documents connected to the role of the laity and the health care mission of the Church, and time for discussion and sharing. The days end with quiet time in Eucharistic Adoration, a meditation on the healing activity of Jesus in the scriptures, reflection, an opportunity for sacramental confession, and a chance to share moments of encouragement and grace in one's role of evangelizing in health care for Christ. What the new evangelization in health care concretely means is leaders sharing with fellow leaders how God has helped them to bring the healing love of Jesus to administrative decisions they made, hiring procedures, budgeting, spiritual comments to staff and talks they've given to fellow leaders, staff, physicians, or patients and their families. A renewed emphasis on sharing their faith in Jesus will assist participants in publicly witnessing to God's increased work in their lives and ministry.

Day One

The first evening allows stressed Catholic health care leaders to unwind and develop a calm spirit before the next day in order to be more able to listen to God. All the leaders are asked to allow the Holy Spirit to guide them on the retreat, to let go of any problems and concerns they are carrying, and to invite God to bring peace to their heart. The goal is for them to hear the loving Shepherd's call: What is he saying to me personally? After the introduction, the leader of the retreat provides a place, ideally a chapel, where the scriptural story of the Good Samaritan from the Gospel of Luke 10:25-37 is read and reflected upon. The leader shares an exegesis or a *lectio divina* (divine reading) on this Gospel passage. The leader should allow for 30 minutes of quiet time with directed questions that reflect on Jesus' role in healing and how leaders can implement the healing ministry of Jesus into their health care ministry. There is an opportunity to share accounts of how their ministry has been like the Good Samaritan's or what their health care facility has done to bring Christ's healing and saving love to those in their care. These moments of sharing allow the health care leaders to see how others have carried out Jesus' healing ministry.

Day Two

Day two is the core of the weekend and includes a morning session, an afternoon session, and an evening session. The goal of this day includes a study of the healing presence of God in the Old Testament, of Jesus' healing in the New Testament, the deeper meaning of healings as recorded by the scriptural authors, and the actual call and responsibility to carry out these works of healing in the world, thus living the call of the new evangelization. As an example of bringing the faith in a new way to Catholic health care leaders, this could be lived out by the Catholic hospital leader making a parish retreat program, or giving a spiritually grounded talk on the meaning of Catholic health care to a Kiwanis club, hosting a pro-life conference for all hospital staff and the public, or sponsoring a parish based community clinic for the poor.

Morning Session

The morning session begins with a brief intro on the history of Catholic health care in the United States. All Catholic health care leaders need to clearly understand the foundation and viewpoint from which they serve today. The Sisters came at the bequest of Church leaders and prominent lay men and women from throughout the world to serve with Christ-like care and compassion the poor, abandoned women and children, the sick, and diseased. Recounting and reflection on what they did, with so little, shows that this ministry is truly the work of God. A complete understanding of this founding will help the leaders see the legacy of those whose footsteps they are following and to continue the passion and care which the Sisters exhibited in their founding hospital or clinic.

The next presentation continues the discussion of religious sponsors and their traditions, e.g., the Mercy Sisters, Franciscans, Sisters of Charity, etc. This topic is important because it helps the leaders to understand the particular reasons for the care they provide at their Catholic health care institution, the particular charisms that inspire the work of their institution, and how this work is carried out throughout their facility. This session also connects the current lay leaders' role within the Church as part of its mission and the role of the Diocesan Bishop in whose name the institution ministers. How can that partnership be enhanced, increased or established. Why is the Bishop's role important for the ministry of Catholic health care in the diocese in which the hospital carries on the mission of Jesus? The focus of Catholic health care as a ministry of the Church is an essential piece of any retreat and is oftentimes glossed over or omitted in formation.

The final portion of the morning is an opportunity for discussion among the leaders about the morning conferences and involves questions like the following: What did God accomplish by his healing miracles? Did he touch the sick alone or were others standing by or those who heard the story afterwards affected? Did Jesus' healing foreshadow a more permanent reality of healing? What do we hope to accomplish by our care, compassion, love, and healing in our institution?

What is my role as the spiritual leader of this Catholic health care institution? Do employees of our health care institution see their work as a job or as a ministry for Christ? Is there work-place spirituality within our conversations, work, and healing? What is to be my relationship with the bishop of this diocese, its pastors, and its churches? How does the Church support me as a leader?

Afternoon Session

The first afternoon session addresses the methods of evangelization and the importance of lay spiritual formation and leadership. It begins with a meditation on Matthew 28:16-20, where Jesus sends the apostles out to continue his ministry of proclaiming the saving Kingdom of God by baptizing, teaching, and making other disciples. It serves to answer the question *why* we are sent and to *whom* we are sent. These are essential questions for Catholic health care leaders to grasp: that Catholic health care is a continuation of Jesus' mission to the sick, the infirm, the poor, the vulnerable, the outcast, the sinner needing salvation, and families needing forgiveness. In other words, as a continuation of the healing ministry of Jesus, Catholic health care is thus a *mission of the Church*. Catholic health care is, we might say, the Gospel message in miniature. Once again, at the end, leaders are given the opportunity to share their testimony of how they have lived this Gospel parable, especially in the context of their institution.

The second afternoon presentation builds on the topic of lay spirituality for leaders by focusing on Ephesians 4:11-12. Only by having a deep dependence on the Holy Spirit can leaders be equipped for ministry. God has given each health care leader a particular gift for the building up of the Church in Catholic health care; that gift must be used, developed, and nurtured so that those who come to experience healing may see this spirit-inspired gift. Hospitals, now led by lay leaders, could experience and see the charisms, inspired by the Holy Spirit, in their previous institution. But now, with the complete departure from leadership or administration of the religious, that charism has mostly vanished. Determining the charism, through some type of *Called & Gifted*[191] program would be essential at this juncture to determine where the spiritual gifts lay for Catholic health care leaders.

Unveiling this Spirit-led gift then helps the lay leaders to respond to the invitation and call that came particularly through the teachings of the Second Vatican Council. Each lay leader, from his or her baptism in Jesus, shares in the prophetic ministry of making Jesus known and loved. They will be called to do this in their daily ministry and work in Catholic health care. Whether that is by leading prayer before every meeting, speaking on a spiritual topic to physicians, attending daily Mass regularly in the Catholic hospital chapel, or myriad other ways, Catholic health care leaders can help promote the new evangelization in such ways.

The third afternoon session focuses on particular passages from *Lumen Gentium* and *Gaudium et Spes,* as well as the *Charter for Healthcare Workers* from the Pontifical Council. These works are read and discussed in detail. Moreover, there is an in-depth study of the most current edition of the *Ethical and Religious Directives for Catholic Healthcare Services.*

The evening session centers on providing the spiritual

---

191 Called and Gifted is a program offered by the charismatic renewal movement of the Catholic Church that seeks to identify and embrace the particular spiritual gifts one has received or utilizes in growing in God's grace and assisting others through this gift of the Holy Spirit.

grounding for living out an evangelizing ministry, first in the life of the lay leader and then in the leader's methods, policies, intentional hiring, forming, and training of future leaders in Catholic health care. If Catholic health care leaders are going to be equipped for ministry, they must be provided with the necessary tools for combatting evil and bringing the presence of Christ to all whom they serve, both partners and patients. If they do not lead so as to make the Gospel of Christ known in their words and actions, then Catholic health care will not be an effective tool for evangelization, and in fact, might even cause scandal to the people of the area.

One of the last sessions each Catholic health care leader will be exposed and guided to reflect upon is the theological understanding of redemptive suffering. This session, using in particular *Salvifici Dolores*, and encyclical by Saint John Paul II, addresses the redemptive and sanctifying meaning of human suffering through Jesus' own passion and explains how Jesus' passion makes sense of one's own suffering. The topic of suffering is very misunderstood today and can truly help people to realize that their ultimate home is in heaven with the Lord. Suffering is part of the imperfect condition caused by sin and so suffering is a way of sharing the redemption wrought be Jesus and sanctification and perfection of one's life.

The last evening session provides an opportunity for Catholic health care leaders to see themselves and their ministry as having a direct effect on furthering the mission of the Church in the world. Leaders are guided to see that Catholic health care is a mission of Jesus to heal, to make whole, and to make the kingdom of God present in the care, love, and healing of those who are sick. One cannot help but be edified by the remark made to Mother Teresa after she picked up and washed one of her first suffering and dying patients. The patient asked her, "Are you Jesus?" How wonderful it would be if patients or the staff of the medical center would say this today! Developing and deepening one's personal relationship with Jesus is essential if our Catholic health care leaders are going to authentically live out the mission of Catholic health care founded by Christ.

Within this session, a presentation is given on the necessary relationship between Catholic health care ministry and the Church, as specifically represented by the Bishop of the local Church. The Bishop is the head of the Church's entire ministry in his diocese and Catholic health care is one of those ministries, along with Catholic schools, Catholic institutions of higher education, and other Catholic entities. The health care leader needs to understand, appreciate, and work with the diocesan bishop. Regular meetings, at least four meetings yearly, are necessary to create the relationship and provide direction and a common understanding of the Church's mission, that is, an understanding from both the bishop's perspective and that of the CEO of the Catholic hospital. Having regular contact will ensure the mission of Catholic health care remains intact and contributes to the unity in Christ within the diocese.

The final presentation provides an opportunity to discuss how Catholic health care can practically partner with Catholic parishes, Catholic grade schools and high schools, Catholic charities, pro-life groups, and Catholic institutions of learning and formation. This outreach into the community extends the message of evangelization and helps the hospital to partner with others in bringing the healing message of Christ to all. It helps the community and the world at large that there is one faith lived in the unity of each Catholic institution.

Finally, the Catholic health care leader should see his or her relationship within the community as a means of promoting the new evangelization. Our Catholic hospitals should be viewed as an extension of Christ's healing presence in the way the entire hospital operates, contributes, functions, cares for, and carries out its mission in Christ. Under this type of leadership, the community, including religious ministers of other denominations and anyone else interested, is invited to the hospital so that they can encounter its Christ-like and compassionate culture. All departments of the hospital, and especially all people engaging in the mission of Catholic health care, should be seen as contributing to this culture of making Christ known by offering care, compassion, joy, peace, patience, and healing to every patient, every time.

The retreat would conclude with a witness presentation from a Catholic health care leader who was able to accomplish many of the goals expressed throughout this retreat. The presenter, having gone through a previous leadership formation program, is a servant leader who makes Jesus' healing known in their own institution and who is striving to advance the mission of the Church through their leadership. Pope Saint Paul VI's quote is very apropos here: "Modern man listens more willingly to witnesses than to teachers, and if he does listen to teachers, it is because they are witnesses."[192]

The day concludes with Eucharistic Adoration.

Retreat Readings

Luke 10:25-37
Matthew 28:16-20

---

192 Pope Paul VI, *Evangelii Nuntiandi*, 41

Ephesians 4:11–12
Lumen Gentium
Gaudium et Spes
Charter for Healthcare Workers from the Pontifical Council
Ethical and Religious Directives for Catholic Healthcare
Services
Salvifici Dolores

Bibliography

Arbuckle, Gerald A. *Catholic Identity or Identities? Refounding Ministries in Chaotic Times.* Collegeville, MN: Liturgical Press, 2013.

Arbuckle, Gerald A. "Maintaining Prophetic Cultures." *Health Progress* (September–October 2005), 19-24.

Archer, David L. "Will Catholic hospitals survive without government reimbursements?" *The Linacre Quarterly* (84) 1, 2017, 23-28.

Ashley, Benedict M. O.P. and Kevin D. O'Rourke O.P. *Healthcare Ethics: A Theological Analysis.* St. Louis, MO: The Catholic Health Association, 1989.

Bechtle, Regina. "Giving the Spirit a Home: Reflections on the Spirituality of Institutions." In *Called & Chosen: Toward a Spirituality for Lay Leaders*, ed. Zeni Fox and Regina Bechtle, 99-111. Lanham, MD: Rowman & Littlefield Publishers, 2005.

Buckeye, Jeanne and Michael Naughton. "The Importance of leadership formation." *Health Progress* (March-April 2008), 38-42.

Casey, Juliana. "Formation for Lay Ministry: Learnings from Religious Life." In *Lay Ecclesial Ministry: Pathways Toward the Future*, ed. Zeni Fox, 143-155.

Chaput, Charles. "The Future of the Catholic Health Care Vocation." *Origins* 39 no. 40, March 18, 2010, 654-658

Chrysostom, John. *Commentary on the Epistle to the Galatians and Homilies on the Epistle to the Ephesians.* A Library of Fathers of the Holy Catholic Church, Anterior to the Division of the East and West. London: Baxter Printer, 1845.

Congregation for the Doctrine of the Faith. *Iunvenescit Ecclesiae* (The Church Rejuvenates), May 15, 2016. On the Relationship between the Hierarchical and Charismatic Gifts in the Life and Mission of the Church. http://www.vatican. va/roman_curia/congregations/cfaith/documents/rc_con_ cfaith_doc_20160516_iuvenescit-ecclesia_en.html (accessed on January 4, 2018).

Congregation for the Doctrine of the Faith. "Some Principles for Collaboration with Non-Catholic Entities in the Provision of Healthcare Services." February 17, 2014 as a response to a letter dated April 15, 2013 from Cardinal Timothy Dolan as President of United States Bishops Conference which presented a *dubium* regarding the transformation of a Catholic health system into a non-Catholic health system.

Delbecq, Andre L. and Jack Mudd and Celeste Mueller. "Formation of Organizational Leaders For Catholic Mission and Identity." *Journal of Jesuit Business Education*, Vol 3, Issue 1, (Summer 2012), 57-73.

Downey, Michael. "'Without a Vision the People Perish: Foundations for a Spirituality of Lay Leadership." In *Called & Chosen: Toward a Spirituality for Lay Leaders*, ed. Zeni Fox and

Regina Bechtle, 17-29. Lanham, MD: Rowman & Littlefield Publishers, 2005.

Dulles, Avery. "The Charism of the New Evangelizer." In *Retrieving Charisms for the Twenty-First Century*, ed. Doris Donnelly, 33-45. Collegeville, MN: The Liturgical Press, 1999.

Gallagher, John A. "Discerning the Future of the American Catholic Health Ministry." *The National Catholic Bioethics Quarterly*, Vol. 13 (2), Summer 2013, 263-274.

Giammalvo, Peter J. "A 'Second Generation' of Ministry Leadership." *Health Progress*, (September–October 2005), 15-18.

Gilden, Lisa. "Exploring Legal Models To Preserve Catholicity." *Health Progress* (May-June 2017), 35-39.

Gormally, Luke. "Pope John Paul's Teaching on Human Dignity and Its Implications for Bioethics." *Philosophy & Medicine* 84 (2012), **7-33**.

Grisez, Germain. Difficult Moral Questions, Vol 3. and "How far may Catholic Hospitals cooperate with providers of immoral services," Question 87. 391-402. Quincy, IL: Franciscan Press, 1997.

Haefs, Lisa. "Laity Look to Preserve Mission of Catholic Health Care." *The Compass: Official Newspaper for the Catholic Diocese of Green Bay, Wisconsin*. February 25, 2015.

Hahnenberg, Edward. "Ordained and Lay Ministry: Restarting the Conversation." *Origins* 35 (6), June 23, 2005, 94-99.

Illinois Hospital Association. "What's at Stake?" 2017. (A

brochure) https://webcache.googleusercontent.com/search?q
=cache:7dgpfV1yULsJ:https://www.team-iha.org/files/non-
gated/advocacy/advocacy-day-message-card.as (accessed on
January 5, 2018).

Kauffman, Christopher J. *Ministry & Meaning: A Religious
History of Catholic Health Care in the United States.* New York,
NY: Crossroad, 1995.

Kee, Howard C. *Medicine, Miracle and Magic in the New
Testament Times.* London: Cambridge University Press, 1986.

Latkovic, Mark S. "The Vocation to Heal: Health Care in
the Light of Catholic Faith: Scriptural, Theological, and
Philosophical Reflections." *The Linacre Quarterly* 75(1), 2008,
40-55.

Lawler, Ronald D. *The Christian Personalism of John Paul II.*
Chicago, IL: Franciscan Herald Press, 1982.

Letourneau, Jim. "Mission Integration and Workplace
Spirituality." *Health Progress* (March-April 2016), 30-32.

Lysaught, M. Therese. *Caritas in Communion: Theological
Foundations of Catholic Health Care.* St. Louis, MO: Catholic
Health Association, 2014.

Lysaught, M. Therese. "Clinically Integrated Networks: A
Cooperation Analysis." *A White Paper.* St. Louis, MO: Catholic
Health Association, 2015.

Martin, Ralph. "A New Pentecost? Catholic Theology and
'Baptism in the Spirit.'" *Logos* 13 (3), Summer 2011.

McGuinness, Margaret M. *Called to Serve: A History of Nuns in America*. New York, NY: New York University Press, 2013.

Merdian, Mark J. "Catholic Health Care Audits." *Ethics & Medics*, 2011, April (36) 4, 1-4.

Minda, Julie. "Dozens of faith-based providers targeted in pension lawsuits." *Catholic Health World*, October 1, 2016.

Mudd, John O. "From CEO to Mission Leader." *Health Progress*, (September–October 2005), 25-27.

Muddiman, John. *The Epistle to the Ephesians*. Grand Rapids, MI: Eerdmans, 1999.

Naumann, Joseph F. "The encounter with the Living God is the foundation of Christian medical practice." *The Linacre Quarterly* 83(3), 2016, 235-238.

Nelson, Leonard J. *Diagnosis Critical: The Urgent Threats Confronting Catholic Health Care*. Huntington, IN: Our Sunday Visitor, 2009.

O'Brien, Peter T. *The Letter to the Ephesians*. Grand Rapids, MI: Eerdmans, 1999.

O'Connell, Lawrence J. and John Shea. *Tradition on the Move: Leadership Formation in Catholic Health Care*. Sacramento, CA: Ministry Leadership Center Press, 2013.

O'Malley, John W. *What Happened at Vatican II*. Cambridge, MA: Harvard University Press, 2008.

O'Rourke, Alice. *The Good Work Begun: Centennial History of Peoria Diocese*. Peoria, IL: The Lakeside Press, 1977.

Pellegrino, Edmund D. and David C. Thomasma. "Charity in Action: Compassion and Caring." In *The Christian Virtues in Medical Practice*, 84-98. Washington, DC: Georgetown University Press, 1996.

Pijnenburg, Martien A. M., Bert Gordijn, Frans J.H. Vosman, and Henk A.M.J. "Catholic Healthcare Organizations and the Articulation of Their Identity." *HEC Forum* (2008), 20 (1), 75-97.

Pontifical Council for Health Care Workers. "Pastoral Care in Health and the New Evangelization for the Transmission of the Faith." Gorle (BG): Editrice VELAR, 2014.

Pope Benedict XVI. *Deus Caritas Est (God is Love,* 2005).

Pope Benedict XVI. *Jesus of Nazareth.* New York, NY: Doubleday, 2007.

Pope Francis. "A Big Heart Open to God: An Interview with Pope Francis." *America* (September 30, 2013). https://www.americamagazine.org/faith/2013/09/30/big-heart-open-god-interview-pope-francis (accessed on October 23, 2017).

Pope Francis. General Audience, March 27, 2013. https://w2.vatican.va/content/francesco/en/audiences/2013/documents/papa-francesco 20130327 udienza-generale.html (accessed February 21, 2018).

Pope Francis. "'Heal the Wounds': Best Practices for the Church as a Field Hospital." *America* (March 4, 2014). https://www.americamagazine.org/issue/%E2%80%98heal-wounds%E2%80%99 (Accessed March 10, 2018).

Pope Francis. Homily at Mass, Cathedral of Sts. Peter and Paul, Philadelphia. Apostolic Journey to the United States, September 26, 2015. https://m.vatican.va/content/francesco/en/homilies/2015/documents/papa-francesco_20150926_usa-omelia-philadelphia.html (accessed November 22, 2017).

Pope Francis. "Message of His Holiness Pope Francis for the Twenty-Sixth World Day of the Sick 2018."

Pope Francis. *The Joy of the Gospel (Evangelii Gaudium)*. Frederick, MD: The Word Among Us Press, 2013.

Pope John XXIII. *Pacem en Terris (Peace on Earth,* 1963).

Pope Paul VI. *Evangelii Nuntiandi (On Proclaiming the Gospel,* 1975)

Pope John Paul II. "Address of His Holiness John Paul II to the Leaders in Catholic Health Care." Phoenix, Arizona, September 14, 1987). http://w2.vatican.va/content/john-paul-ii/en/speeches/1987/september/documents/hf_jp-ii_spe_19870914_organiz-sanitarie-cattoliche.html (accessed on January 14, 2018).

Pope John Paul II. "Address to the Catholic Health Association," (September 14, 1987). http://w2.vatican.va/content/john-paul-ii/en/speeches/1987/september/documents/hf_jp-ii_spe_19870914_organiz-sanitarie-cattoliche.html (accessed on January 23, 2018).

Pope John Paul II. *Dolentium Hominum* (Apostolic Letter establishing the Pontifical Commission for the Apostolate of Health Care Workers, 1985).

Pope John Paul II. *Evangelium Vitae* (*The Gospel of Life*, 1995).

Pope John Paul II. "Letter to Families," (February 2, 1994). https://w2.vatican.va/content/john-paul-ii/en/letters/1994/documents/hf_jp-ii_let_02021994_families.html (accessed on January 4, 2018)

Pope John Paul II. "Opening Address to the Assembly of CELAM." Port-au-Prince, Haiti, March 9, 1983 (translation from *L'Osservatore Romano* English Edition 16/780, April 18, 1983, no. 9).

Pope John Paul II. *Redemptoris Missio (The Mission of the Redeemer*, 1990).

Pope John Paul II. *Veritatis Splendor* (The Splendor of Truth, 1993).

Pope Pius XII. "Address to an International Congress of Anesthesiologists." November 24,1957. http://www.lifeissues.net/writers/doc/doc_31resuscitation.html (accessed on January 5, 2018).

Popovici, Alice. "Shift to laity sparks formation needs." *National Catholic Reporter*. February 21, 2012.

Ratzinger, Joseph. *Theological Highlights of Vatican II*. New York: Paulist Press, 1966.

Rohlfs, Steven. "Dye, Not Paint: Issues in Catholic Identity." *Ethics & Medics* (February 1997) 22(2), 1-2.

Rohlfs, Steven. "The Experience of Catholic Health Care." *Ethics & Medics* (February 1997) 22(2), 3-4.

Schall, James V. "Will Catholic Hospitals be the Next Target?" *Crisis*, September 1, 2015.

Schmiesing, Kevin. "A History of Personalism." Unpublished manuscript. May 26, 2011. https://papers.ssrn.com/sol3/papers.cfm?abstract_id=1851661

Second Vatican Council. *Ad Gentes* (Decree on the Missionary Activity of the Church, 1965).

Second Vatican Council. *Apostolicam Acousitatem* (Decree on the Apostolate of the Laity, 1965).

Second Vatican Council. *Gaudium et Spes* (Pastoral Constitution on the Church in the Modern World, 1965).

Second Vatican Council. *Lumen Gentium* (Dogmatic Constitution on the Church, 1964).

_____. "The Light Obscured: Mis-insurance and a Missing Relationship, Healthcare in America: A Catholic Proposal for Renewal." A statement of the Catholic Medical Association, September, 2004. http://www.cathmed.org/assets/files/CMA%20Healthcare%20Task%20Force%20Statement%209.04%20Website.pdf (accessed on February 23, 2018).

Shaw, Russell. *Ministry or Apostolate: What Should the Catholic Laity Be Doing?* Huntington: Our Sunday Visitor, 2002.

Smith, Brian P. and Patricia Talone. "Preliminary Results: CHA Survey Gauges Formation Effectiveness." *Health Progress* (July–August 2014), 44-49.

Stanley, Teresa. "Can the Ministry Collaborate to Form the

'Next Generation' of Sponsors?" *Health Progress* (January-February 2007), 12-15.

Sulmasy, Daniel P. "Without Love, We Perish: Gospel-Centered Health Care Is a Radical Approach in Today's Secular World." *Health Progress* (July–August 2009), 30-36.

The National Catholic Bioethics Center. *New Charter for Health Care Workers.* Philadelphia: NCBC, 2017.

The New York Times. "The White House Puts the Bible Before the Hippocratic Oath," by The Editorial Board, January 28, 2018.

United States Conference of Catholic Bishops. *The Ethical and Religious Directives for Catholic Health Care Services*, Fifth Edition, 2009. Washington, DC.

United States Conference of Catholic Bishops Committee on Evangelization and Catechesis. *Living as Missionary Disciples.* Washington, D.C.: USCCB Publishing, 2017.

Uttley, Lois and Sheila Reynertson. "The Growth of Catholic Hospitals and the Threat to Reproductive Healthcare." *Merger Watch of the American Civil Liberties Union*, New York, NY: Merger Watch, 2013.

Williams, Thomas D. and Jan O. Bengtsson. "Personalism." In *Stanford Encyclopedia of Philosophy.* https://plato.stanford.edu/entries/personalism/ (accessed on January 4, 2018).

Williamson, Peter S. *Ephesians.* Grand Rapids, MI: Baker Academic, 2009.

Made in the USA
Monee, IL
11 January 2020